KEEPING THEM HEALTHY, KEEPING THEM HOME

ELLEN M. CARUSO, R.N.

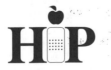

HEALTH INFORMATION PRESS

Los Angeles, California 90010

Library of Congress Cataloging-in-Publication Data

Caruso, Ellen M., 1965-
    Keeping them healthy, keeping them home : how to care for your loved
ones at home / Ellen M. Caruso.
        p. cm.
    Includes index.
    ISBN 1-885987-13-7
    1. Home care services. 2. Home nursing. 3. Caregivers.
I. Title
RA645.3.C376 1998   98-26957
362.1'4--dc21   CIP

ISBN: 1-885987-13-7

Health Information Press
4727 Wilshire Blvd.
Los Angeles, CA 90010
1-800-MED-SHOP
http://www.medicalbookstore.com

Printed in the United States of America

This publication is designed to provide accurate and authoritative information
regarding the subject matter covered. It is sold with the understanding that the
publisher and author are not engaged in rendering professional advice or services.
The information contained herein is solely the opinion of the author. Though all of
the information contained herein has been carefully checked and researched for
accuracy and completeness, neither the author nor the publisher accept any liability
or responsibility with regard to errors, omissions, misuse, or misinterpretation.

DEDICATION

"Never may the flaw consume the vessel"

*This book is dedicated to all who contribute to patient care at home,
from family to volunteers to professional staff—every effort makes a difference.
To the patients who have so graciously accepted me into their homes and
therefore their lives: Thank you.*

AUTHOR'S NOTE

The information presented in this text is strictly a result of my professional experience as a registered nurse. Patients I have visited or cared for over the last twelve years have all unknowingly contributed to the writing of this book. No one individual can be singled out for individual reference nor are any specific case examples presented. The only source used in compiling this information was in the listing of abbreviations that is used by my employer of the past seven years for reference within the agency. The abbreviations are all medically accepted and widely use by any medical personnel so this information can not be claimed by any individual or group as being their own or original. Comments to the author are welcome via e-mail: Emctc@aol.com or visit my website: http://members.aol.com/Emctc/index.html.

ACKNOWLEDGEMENTS

Special thanks to:

My parents for not only giving me wings, but for teaching me how to fly.

Garry Feldman of U. S. Computer Connection, Stamford, CT who technically made it all possible.

Cheryl Ciofalo, who personifies endurance and resilience: shine on.

Renata, for her grace, excitement, love an support.

Cochran School of Nursing and St. Johns Riverside Hospital of Yonkers, NY who care for the person as well as the patient.

Tommy, Michael and Jimmy, for teaching me survival skills.

Dr. Doreen Virtue, author and mentor and true angel.

Home Nursing Association of Westchester, for their dedication to quality patient care.

TJ and Stephen for 7:30 bedtimes.

Kathryn Swanson, Editor and Pamela Parker, Marketing Director of Health Information Press, and Kate Bandos of KSB Promotions for graciously doing the lion's share of work that brought this book into your hands.

And mostly to Tom, for his humor, warmth and love.

TABLE OF CONTENTS

PREFACE

Patients are leaving the hospital "sicker and quicker" as the advent of managed care has reduced coverage for hospital stays. The introduction of Diagnostic Related Groupings (DRGs) and other patient assessment tools has reduced the amount of time that a patient may remain in the hospital. Under these programs, each diagnosis has a number of days assigned to it, which reflects the maximum number of hospital days for which an insurance company will pay. For patients with several diagnoses or who have complications during a hospital stay, the number of allowable days may be extended if the need is justified.

In addition, modern medicine has reduced many complications of the natural aging process leaving an elderly population to care for themselves, often with concerns that require intervention but not constant medical treatment.

Home health care fills the gap between discharge from the hospital and the patient's full recovery from illness. The patient that is referred for home care from the hospital will be sent home with a list of current treatments and instructions regarding when to follow up with the doctor. This is only a small amount of the information needed to allow the patient to recover to his fullest ability and reduce re-admission. Use of skilled nursing visits to the patient at home can also provide patient education regarding treatments, diagnosis and medications that would produce costly hospital bills if done prior to discharge.

Home care agencies also help plan patient care for the future. The planning involves education and intervention regarding the medical or social problems that are identified by the visiting nurse. The inability of the home care team to teach about every possible situation that may arise for a patient—whether due to insurance limitations on visits, time constraints or the human inability to absorb and retain large quantities of information, especially when under stress—is what prompted the writing of this book.

Caregivers are often adult children who are sandwiched between the needs of their own children and spouse, and those of their parent. Proximity to the patient, work obligations and personal needs reduce the time that the caregiver can physically spend coordinating and actively participating in the patient's home care. This book offers a comprehensive approach to assessing the patient's physical needs and living environment, and realistic solutions for meeting the needs that are identified.

It also offers practical information that is hard to find anywhere else. Caregivers without any previous health or medical knowledge can use this book as a guide in providing and overseeing safe and effective patient care. For example, insurance companies and hospitals have found it cost effective to align themselves with home care agencies and medical equipment suppliers. Some insurance companies are exclusive or contracted in their use of both types of health care providers. A patient needs to be aware of such alliances if making his own referral for home care. When a home care agency receives a patient referral, it will research the patient's insurance to determine if any restrictions apply to the frequency of visits or if use of ancillary services might be approved. If the patient is eligible for home care through a contract agency only, the staff member will advise the patient who can then contact the approved provider.

Other topics range from how to obtain home care services, through death and dying at home with practical information and resources. Formal and informal caregivers will find that the use of preventative measures facilitates a healthier patient and therefore reduces hospitalization and the onset of new health concerns. However, this book is meant only as a *guide* for home health care. As each person is unique, so are their health care needs. The doctor is always the guiding force when implementing a plan to meet the patient's needs and should be consulted accordingly.

1

OBTAINING HOME CARE SERVICES

Upon the patient's discharge from the hospital or health care facility, a referral for a home care service evaluation can be made by the discharge planner. The doctor approves the referral by agreeing to be responsible for orders while the patient is receiving home care. Physician involvement may include discussion with the patient's primary nurse or other members of the home care agency, and approving changes in the plan of care.

The discharge planner should explain the care and support that will be needed at home along with possible resources for assistance before making a home care referral. If home care is suggested in the hospital, but the family or caregiver does not feel that this is an option, they need to communicate this to the discharge planner so alternate plans can be made.

For patients who are admitted to the hospital and have had prior home care services, the discharge planner may assume that this will be the plan for discharge. When patient care becomes more involved, or when patients have a change in their ability to care for themselves, the previous caregivers should ask what changes in supervision and involvement may be needed. The best plan for post-hospital care is the one that meets the patient's needs at the time of discharge.

Caregivers sometimes have changes in their own needs or abilities that no longer allow them to care for the patient at home. A social worker or pastoral counselor can meet with caregivers to help them sort out the emotions involved when they realize they are unable to take a patient home for care as they had done in the past.

A friend, family or community member may also refer a patient for home care services. The primary doctor will be contacted and made aware of the request for nursing evaluation and at that time agrees to sign medical orders for care. The doctor will review the patient information that is obtained with the referral and may choose to add treatments or clarify medications.

Patients that may benefit from home care services are those with newly diagnosed medical conditions or those with chronic illness that become unstable and therefore have changes in their treatment plans periodically. Patients who are suffering from general effects of the aging process may also benefit from home intervention.

The assessment of each patient to receive skilled nursing care at home is largely a determination of their current medical status, medical history of past and current illness, treatments and interventions. The patient's response to interventions; the ability of the patient or caregiver to learn and retain information regarding the disease process, medications and treatments; and signs of reoccurrence of illness are also assessed.

PAPERWORK

Admission to receive care from a home care agency requires a signed release by the patient or her advocate. This allows the agency to provide service, bill the insurance, and hold the patient responsible for payment of non-covered services. The patient should read this release carefully and be given a copy of it for her records.

The patient may also be asked if she has an advanced directive, which is a living will or health care proxy. The advent of such documents has given patients the ability to prepare in advance for long-term health care and consider their options regarding the interventions they may desire to prolong their lives. These directives assign the responsibility to make decisions about the patient's health care to a specific person in the event that the patient is no longer able to make her own decisions. An attorney specializing in elder law can provide more information regarding this process. The patient will be asked to provide a copy of her directive if it is in effect and it will be kept with the patient record. A copy should also be given to the doctor and to the hospital if admitted so the wishes of the patient are known and respected. Some patients have informally communicated this information to their doctors, but legal application varies state to state. A formal directive on file is more binding.

Table 1.1: Basic Home Care Information
_____

Referral to home care may be made by:
- Hospital discharge planner
- Hospital social worker
- Doctor
- Friend or family member
- Patient

A home care agency can be located through:
- Phone book yellow pages under "Nursing Services"
- Doctor's recommendation of a particular agency
- Local Office of the Aging
- Word of mouth

Nursing services include but are not limited to:
- Physical exam
- Instruction of prescribed medications and treatment regime
- Instruction in disease process, signs and symptoms of alteration in condition that may require doctor notification or emergency intervention
- Performing treatments on a regularly scheduled basis such as wound care, prescribed medication injection
- Identifying safety concerns and implementing a plan to correct them
- Coordination of ancillary service referral

Ancillary services include:
- Physical Therapy (PT)
- Occupational Therapy (OT)
- Speech Therapy (ST)
- Social Worker (SW)
- Home Health Aid (HHA)
- Durable Medical Equipment (DME)
- Home Intravenous Therapy (IVT)
- Laboratory Services

_____

PATIENT CONFIDENTIALITY

On admission to home care services, the nurse will need to know the names of significant others, and who is to be contacted in case of an emergency. This information is part of the patient record. The patient has a right to privacy, and the information recorded by the nurse initially and on subsequent visits is confidential.

Patient charts are usually kept in locked file cabinets in the home care agency and are used by the nurses who visit to record patient status. Records are returned to the office after visits are complete and usually are not left in locations where any non-involved parties can access them.

Members of the health care team actively involved in patient care will share information, but professional ethics prevent discussing patient information with those not directly involved. This practice becomes especially important when caring for the patient at home because health care providers are often seen by neighbors as they visit. By maintaining patient confidentiality, caregivers do not divulge any information to even the most well-meaning neighbors.

THE HOME CARE AGENCY

Home care agencies may be hospital based and employ staff through the hospital, or they may be independent companies. The agency may have its own administrative staff or share it with the parent company. Generally, the agency will have an administrative staff who may or may not have health backgrounds. There is an increasing tendency to have agency directors with business backgrounds instead of medical backgrounds.

In most agencies, a director of nursing presides over the supervisory staff, who in turn are responsible for all team members. Each supervisor may have a separate area of concern—such as nursing or physical therapy—or they may have members from each discipline report to them. Regardless of the structure, the health care providers that visit the patient are responsible to the supervisors and utilize them as a tool when establishing a patient care plan.

The visiting nurse's initial visit may last up to two hours while the patient is assessed and a plan for care is determined. The nurse will decide the frequency of visits that the patient needs and will support the frequency with any paperwork that is mandated by the agency. The nurse will request ancillary services as needed and approved, and will notify the proper department(s). That department and its supervisor are then responsible to assign patients for care to the proper ancillary service provider in a timely manner.

Subsequent visits by the visiting nurse are aimed at fulfilling the plan for instruction and treatment, and monitoring vital signs such as blood pressure, heart and lung function along with a continued assessment of other affected body systems.

The visiting nurse is not meant to bathe or feed the patient during the visit. If the need for such activities arises during the course of the visit, the nurse may do so on a limited basis and then establish a plan for additional services to meet those needs in the future. For example, if the nurse is assessing an area of the patient's body that becomes soiled during the exam, the nurse will assist the caregiver in cleaning the patient.

Team Approach

All health care providers who are involved in a patient's care communicate periodically to address patient-specific issues and needs, and to institute any plan changes. This allows coordination of care and a team approach to the patient. For example, if a therapist feels the patient is experiencing excessive pain during therapy sessions, the therapist may discuss this concern with the home care nurse who may discuss this with the doctor, who may alter pain medication dose or frequency. Additionally if those involved feel that a patient is recovering faster or slower than anticipated, they may jointly discuss how each aspect of the home care team can assist the efforts or alter the plan to allow the patient more independence.

Per Diem Employees

Home care agencies often employ per diem or contract nurses and therapists. These providers are given orientation according to agency policy and must meet the same job requirements regarding quality of patient care as the full-time staff.

Per diem employees are used by an agency to meet staffing needs during vacations, or to supplement staffing when the agency has a large roster of patients. They are responsible to supervisory and administrative staff, and have agency requirements for ongoing inservices and certifications. When using per diem staff, the agency will generally assign the same per diem member to a patient, just as they would a staff member, to offer continuity of care. The patient may become confused or upset if visited by many different providers.

Accreditation

Home care agencies are surveyed on a regular basis to assess that they meet state guidelines for providing patient care. Each agency can provide a list of mandatory and voluntary accreditations that it has received. All surveys for accreditation involve detailed records assessment, and the surveying agency makes actual visits to several patients' homes with a nurse or therapist. A home care agency that applies for and undergoes voluntary accreditations beyond those required by insurance companies or state regulations are generally agencies that are well run and concerned about providing efficient care. This is a way for the agency to assure its clients that they are concerned with meeting patient needs.

SPECIAL NEEDS THAT CAN BE MET BY A HOME CARE AGENCY

Each patient's needs are unique and services are provided accordingly. For example, agencies are often able to provide nurses who are fluent in foreign languages or sign language, or translators if necessary.

Children

When the patient is a child, the agency may provide nurses who have specific pediatric experience. Caregivers may request that the patient be referred to an agency that specializes in pediatric care and/or one that contracts with ancillary providers of pediatric care. Every effort will be made to provide child-sized equipment or personalize items to accommodate the child. Considerations such as schooling and a child's specific socialization needs can be discussed with involved parties and a social worker referred as needed. Counseling may be necessary or welcome for families and caregivers of children with terminal illnesses. Generally a child who is terminally ill is cared for by a medical institution that is familiar with local agencies that can provide pediatric home care. The national organization for a specific disease may also be familiar with community resources for pediatric patients.

Every effort will be made to maintain the normalcy of this patient's routine because of the negative impact that disruption of routines can have on a child's development, emotional balance, and response to medical intervention. The needs of the parents and caregivers are also given special consideration, especially when other children live in the home. The effort to maintain normalcy is extremely important so the child does not feel that he is disrupting the family. The child's ability to recognize his impact on the rest of the family should not be underestimated.

It is further not unusual for other children in the family to feel resentment that the ill child is receiving extra attention. Spending separate time with each child is important if possible. Bookstores have a selection of children's books aimed at dealing with illness of family and friends, and also with death.

More Than One Patient

Another unique home care situation is when two family members are ill and require service, or when one becomes ill while the other is under home nursing care. In this situation, every effort is made to involve other family or friends in care. Parts of the patient's care may be provided by home health aids for personal needs, and emergency systems for ambulance access may be implemented. The use of home delivered meals can reduce cooking needs.

If both family members are insured by the same plan, the insurance company may combine home health aid time and increase the allowance, or have the same aid stay for concurrent hours. The home care agency can assist with scheduling solutions that meet the patient's needs and the insurance company's restrictions.

When a primary caregiver becomes the patient—for example, the husband who was responsible for the spouse's care and household upkeep such as grocery shopping—the care plan may be based on the caregiver's potential for recovery and resumption of his previous role. The doctor will be involved in determining the level of rehabilitation anticipated. If it appears that the primary caregiver will not be able to resume patient care after he recovers, a plan on how to best care for both people will be made with the involvement of family or an advocate. If neither exist, the discharge planner may make plans for one or both of the patients to go to a facility that can meet their needs. The doctor will be involved in making these plans. An agency such as an adult protective may also be involved in establishing the most effective plan in this situation.

Skilled Care

Some patients require highly skilled care or extensive hands-on personal care. This would apply, for example, to patients who are mechanically ventilated at home, usually through a tracheostomy. The tracheostomy is an artificial opening in the trachea that allows for the patient to receive the oxygen he needs to live. The ventilator is the means by which the patient breathes.

This type of patient needs many aspects of care and many supporting pieces of equipment, such as suction machines and the ventilator itself. Adequate room in the patient's environment along with electrical outlets in close proximity to the patient are required. Additionally, the caregiver must be able to learn all aspects of care, from cleaning the tracheostomy tube that is in the patient's throat, suctioning the patient's tracheostomy and using emergency procedures if the trachea becomes blocked. The caregiver must be taught to recognize and respond rapidly to symptoms and signs. This patient can never be left unattended, or in the care of a person who is not fully aware of the patient's needs and of appropriate emergency responses. Registered nurses are available for skilled home care on a shift basis.

Comatose patients may also be cared for in the home if adequate caregivers are available. The specific needs for this type of patient will be discussed prior to discharge from the hospital since each patient's needs are unique. It may include feeding tubes, urinary drainage tubes as well as routine skin care to prevent breakdown.

Any patient with such involved needs will be carefully considered before becoming a candidate for home care. Assessment of the caregivers' abilities and their understanding of the extent of the patient's needs will be done. The need for supplemental caregivers will be made clear. Patients that require extensive care are not prohibited from obtaining home care services if their needs can be met safely.

2

SERVICES AVAILABLE AT HOME

NURSING

A registered nurse will make an evaluation visit after the home care agency receives a referral for care. The referral includes basic insurance information, personal data such as birth date, address, doctor's name, diagnosis, current medication, and planned referral services.

A referral that is received by the home care agency from a friend or family member is commonly called a community referral. The patient's doctor is contacted for approval of the initial visit and agrees to provide orders for home care services with availability for involvement in patient care.

A patient who is discharged from the hospital is referred to a home care agency by the social worker, discharge planner, or doctor. The information provided from a hospital discharge referral is more extensive, often including copies of consultations, lab test results, medications used in the hospital, and the patient's progress during his hospital stay. The hospital referral will identify people involved in the patient's care and any instructions they were given prior to discharge.

This referral information will give the nurse an idea of the patient's immediate needs so that a plan can start to be formed even before the patient is seen at home. An example of this may be a patient who will require daily injections of medication, or daily wound care. The nurse can anticipate some of the medical supplies and services that will be needed, and can order them before the first nursing visit at home.

Despite receiving personal and insurance information on a referral, the nurse will actually need to see any insurance cards, and confirm birth date, Social Security number and the correct spelling of the patient's name. This helps make the billing more efficient, and can clarify if the insurance is in the patient's own name or the spouse's name.

Initially, the nurse will assess the patient's physical status, performing a complete physical even if the patient was referred for a specific problem. The nurse must evaluate all patients, even if they clearly have a need for ancillary services only. This helps to identify the patient's general health and potential response to care, and it may uncover other medical needs that could benefit from intervention. For example, a person with a wound will also need nutritional instruction as proper eating habits will aid healing.

The initial assessment will include a review of current medications. The nurse will want to know which ones are new, if any are replacements for old medications, and if there were any changes in frequency, dose or route.

An evaluation of the home environment for unsafe or unhealthy conditions will be made at this time. This does not mean that the nurse will be prying into the patient's personal belongings. She will be assessing whether there is adequate food, electricity, and telephone services available.

An assessment of the patient's ability to learn and the availability of additional teachable persons who could be caregivers will also be made. At this point, the nurse may identify the primary caregiver and others who will take part in patient care.

Relationships within families all vary, as do family members' abilities and desires to participate in patient care. From the beginning of patient care, the nurse needs to be aware of the extent to which family members will be involved. In trying to determine this, the nurse will ask questions. In so doing, she is not expecting family members to provide patient care simply because they are related, and is not passing judgment on lack of family interest in regards to the patient. The nurse knows that the situation she finds may not be a true indication of how the family functioned in the past; a patient that is pleasant and cooperative towards the nurse may not have been this way towards the family. In any case, the patient's family does not need to justify to the nurse or any other health care provider their lack of involvement in patient care.

The sum of the nurse's evaluation is used to establish a plan of care for the patient that will include how often the nurse needs to visit, what goals or outcomes can be expected, and which if any ancillary services will be needed. The plan will help determine whom the nurse will be teaching and what the patient needs to learn in order to maintain or improve his current level of health and functioning.

The initial instruction often deals with the patient's disease process, its effects on the body, and how to recognize signs and symptoms of a worsened condition. Correct time, dose, frequency, use, and potential side effects of medications will be taught, and the nurse will recommend ways to establish a safe administration regime. The nurse will also offer suggestions for making the home environment safe if necessary. There is not a formula for determining the frequency of skilled nursing visits and the original plan may be modified if the patient responds differently than anticipated or if caregiver participation changes.

A plan for care is written in chart-style format that varies according to agency and state guidelines. This chart is a communication tool for each nurse who may visit the patient. Follow-up visits usually do not require the same amount of information gathering as the initial visit, but previously noted details may need clarification.

Patients will be discharged from skilled home care when they are either independent enough to care for themselves, or they have caregivers in place who understand and can perform this care. Some insurance programs limit the frequency of nursing visits, the duration of care and the use of ancillary services. Most managed care programs have some type of restrictions, but offer case-by-case consideration of needs and allowable services. A case manager is usually assigned by the insurance company and the nurse will report the findings and plans for nursing care and ancillary services to that person. Any changes or additions to the patient's care must be approved by the case manager. A breach in following these guidelines may result in non-coverage of services, so it is important for the nurse and patient to be aware of the policy limitations and allowances. It is the responsibility of the nurse and the agency to understand the patient's insurance, but grievances regarding length of service or denial of ancillary services are ultimately the responsibility of the patient or their advocate.

All home care services can be continued with private billing to the patient after insurance coverage ends. If a patient continues to need bathing assistance three times a week, she may prefer to continue with the home health aide who was providing that service from the home care agency. Likewise, the patient may want the physical therapist to continue to help him perform his exercise program, even after being thoroughly instructed and knowledgeable. Many agencies provide sliding scales for fees. There are also occasions where an agency might have grant money or donations available in a fund to provide reduced rates for patients who no longer qualify for insurance-covered services but are unable to meet their own needs unassisted. It is possible for families to make anonymous donations to pay for non-covered services that can reduce a patients sense of dependency.

ANCILLARY SERVICES

Physical Therapy

A physical therapist (PT) is referred by the nurse to evaluate and treat the patient's mobility needs or deficits. The physical therapist's goal is to increase the patient's level of function of the affected muscle groups and/or limb(s) if possible, or instruct the patient in how to maintain current function. The PT will assess the patient's past and current level of functioning, activity tolerance and use of assisting devices, then a program for rehabilitation will be formed. The PT will initiate a plan of exercises, which will be adapted specifically to the patient and take the patient's level of independence, caregiver support and home environment into consideration.

A physical therapist makes a plan for visit frequency independent of the nurse's plan. The PT will try to visit as often as needed, however the patient's insurance coverage may again influence the frequency of visits. The patient is often discharged from physical therapy when his level of function has reached a plateau or a maximum level of function. Sometimes, a PT may plan to resume care in the future after a pivotal point in the patient's progress, such as after a cast is removed or after surgery.

Each plan for therapy is made specific to the patient. It will take into account such circumstances as the patient's motivation, his understanding of instruction (both verbal and by demonstration), and the availability of caregivers. A PT will recommend medical equipment and order it for the patient if insurance allows, or inform the caregiver where it may be purchased.

The nurse who is responsible for the patient's care (usually the admitting nurse) will take a report from the PT regarding the patient's status and response to therapy. The PT will communicate findings, plan for care and the patient's response to specific exercises or treatments.

The doctor may recommend that home physical therapy be discontinued and refer the patient for outpatient physical therapy if the patient's strength improves, or if specific exercise machines at the outpatient facility would be beneficial to the patient.

Occupational Therapy

The occupational therapist (OT) provides the fine tuning for the patient's participation in daily activities. The OT may provide instruction on getting into and out of the bathtub, getting dressed, or preparing meals. He will also provide a customized plan, re-evaluate the plan, and contact the case managing nurse and doctor to advise of patient progress and needs.

The OT is instrumental in suggesting bathroom equipment, tools such as grabbers and reachers for accessing fallen or hard to reach objects, and products to assist with feeding and meal preparation. The OT helps the patient adapt to his own environment with consideration of his needs, physical abilities and limitations.

Speech Therapy

A speech therapist (ST) is referred to assist a patient with communication or oral disabilities such as swallowing. The ST evaluates the patient, determines his needs that can be addressed, and communicates these findings to the doctor and case managing nurse.

The ST's plan will often include exercises for the patient that are done alone or with verbal cues from a caregiver. The patient may need supervision with exercises that focus on swallowing if aspiration is a concern.

Social Worker

A social worker (SW or MSW) is referred by a nurse to evaluate the patient's support system (both formal and informal), to assist with long-term plans, and to offer information regarding community services. The SW will work to involve caregivers in patient needs if they are available and agreeable. If there is not an informal support system or if the patient has areas of dependence that cannot be met through caregivers, the social worker can offer solutions.

Names and numbers for local groceries that deliver, medical alert systems and community elder programs are just a very small example of the services that exist to meet home care needs. Many of the referrals for outside care are made by the social worker him/herself, with the patient's approval. The SW contacts the doctor to discuss the plan of care and relies on input from the doctor and visiting nurse for their impressions of the patient's needs.

The social worker's responsibility is to address the patient's needs and help create a safe and effective plan to meet those needs. The SW is not referred to judge personal relationships or to force family and friends to provide care that they are not willing or able to do.

A social worker may need to recommend inpatient care if the patient cannot be cared for safely or effectively at home. The decision for placement is not made by the SW, but may be discussed with the patient, family or advocate, doctor, and case managing nurse.

Home Health Aid

A home health aid (HHA) is referred by the admitting nurse to assist the patient with his or her personal care. The HHA is trained to provide such care, and home care agencies usually have protocols regarding ongoing inservice education to enhance the HHA skills.

Home health aid service is ordered for a specific number of hours per day, days per week, and weeks at a time. The hours and number of days may taper as the patient becomes more independent in self care.

A specific plan of care is established for the patient. This may include bathing, dressing, bathroom assistance, grooming and ambulation. The HHA may also be involved in the patient's home exercise program if ordered by the nurse and instructed by either the PT, OT, or nurse. The HHA will be supervised by the case managing nurse or advocate on a regular basis.

The hours allowed for HHA care may be dictated by the insurance company. Many home care agencies are able to set up additional HHA hours with separate billing to the patient for those hours that are not covered by insurance. Insurance plans may not be generous with the amount of hours, days and weeks of HHA care. This economy of time is sometimes the hardest part of home care for the patient to understand because the HHA services are often the most needed.

The case managing nurse may be able to explain from the start of care what coverage can be expected from the insurance company regarding length and frequency of HHA services. The nurse or home care agency may be able to offer alternatives for financing or providing care when coverage ends. A social worker may also be referred to offer suggestions or solutions.

The case managing nurse may recommend that a patient have HHA coverage for up to 24 hours a day in cases where there is not a family or friend available to stay with the patient, and the patient is dependent on others for most aspects of care. When this situation occurs and the patient or families refuse or cannot finance these services, the agency may have to refuse to provide all home care services unless a reasonable solution is found. An example is a bedbound patient who is not able to communicate or is unable to access the phone. Because she would not be able to contact emergency services if needed, she would be considered unsafe at home. By having family, friends, or paid caregivers present 24 hours a day, this case would be rectified. Another case would be a patient who is fully ambulatory but has a diagnosis such as Alzheimer's disease. This patient may wander away from the home, leave the gas from the stove on, or become confused if an emergency occurred and be unable to access help. Each patient's individual needs and abilities are assessed, and plans are established and revised so that their needs can be met safely and economically.

If arranging for a 24-hour home health aid, that person must have a place to sleep, and be provided with bathroom facilities and food. The person does not require separate facilities and should arrange for their own food if following restricted or preferred diet. If a patient requires constant care or supervision, two 12-hour home health aids must be used; a 24-hour HHA is expected to receive eight hours of sleep time.

DURABLE MEDICAL EQUIPMENT

Medical equipment includes hospital beds, wheelchairs, walkers, canes, crutches, overbed tables, bed rails, oxygen delivery systems and a variety of others. This group of equipment is usually rented to the patient with varying insurance coverage depending on justification from the doctor and supporting medical documents. Some rentals may convert to sales of the equipment depending on length of use, patient status, insurance coverage and equipment dealer policy.

Another group of medical supplies is bathroom equipment. These items may include bedside commodes, over the toilet commodes, bath seats and bath rails. These items are generally sale-only items because of hygiene reasons, but there are always exceptions and insurance coverage varies. The above items are sometimes sold used through newspaper ads so it is important to know the insurance coverage before agreeing to purchase them new.

A third category of equipment is soft supplies that include dressing supplies, underpads, and adult briefs among others. Underpads and briefs are covered under some plans or can be purchased through general pharmacy services. Cost comparison may determine the best option. Consider any discounts for purchasing in bulk. The nurse who admits the patient for home care services will order any needed supplies usually through a vendor agency with which the home care agency contracts. Supplies that are not covered by insurance but are still needed (often underpads or briefs) may be ordered by the home care agency but paid for by the patient. Each agency will have its own policy regarding this situation.

If a physical therapist or occupational therapist recommends a specific piece of equipment, they will order it or advise the case manager of the need. Any financial responsibility to the patient will be discussed prior to placing the order. Some pieces of bathroom equipment, such as tub rails, need to be permanently installed and the therapist should have a person to recommend for the job.

Once a package of soft supplies is opened and some of the content used, it is not able to be returned for partial credit. Items that are ordered and never used may be able to be returned or exchanged. The policy of the home care agency, insurance, and vendor agency can provide that information. This is an important part of cost containment for insurance companies because in cases of wound care management, supplies may be changed rather frequently.

The vendor agency makes its own arrangements for delivery of equipment and is responsible for the maintenance of it. The managing nurse can intervene on the patient's behalf in some situations to expedite delivery, or to request specifically adapted equipment. Patients will receive an invoice on delivery which should be kept for reference.

Oxygen Therapy

Oxygen therapy is available at home and must be ordered for the patient by the doctor. The doctor will order the amount of oxygen to be administered by indicating the number of liters per minute (lpm), the delivery route (nasal prongs or mask) and the number of hours per day the patient should wear the oxygen with allowances at times for "as needed" (prn) use. An oxygen order may read "O2 at 2 lpm via nasal cannula for twelve hours while sleeping and two to three hours prn during day for shortness of breath unrelieved with rest."

The medical supply company will deliver the oxygen system, explain its correct use and instruct in the care of the system. The patient may receive refills of oxygen at scheduled intervals if using the common liquid oxygen system, or may receive an oxygen concentrator, which is a machine that needs to be plugged in to an electrical outlet and takes room air into the system and returns it to the patient at a purer concentration. The medical supplier will provide a standard oxygen tank for use if the patient leaves the home or in case of power failure when the primary system is a concentrator. Local electric companies should be notified of oxygen use by way of a concentrator so that they can provide a generator for loss of electricity.

Liquid oxygen systems have a smaller portable system that can be filled from the main tank if the patient needs oxygen to leave home. Liquid tanks have gauges to monitor the level of oxygen in the tank and the supplier will advise at which level the refill is needed. General rules for oxygen systems regardless of type are to keep the system and any tubing away from flames or potential fire contact; to turn off the system when it's not in use; and to wash or change the filter in a concentrator as indicated in the instruction book, and care for humidity reservoir if used. The information should be given to the patient orally and in writing by the technician who delivers the system.

The medical supplier's name and phone number must be clearly indicated, as well as a phone number for after-hours service. Many oxygen suppliers employ respiratory therapists who visit the patient after the system has been delivered and will assess for proper use.

Patients should never wear oxygen in the kitchen in the presence of open flames. Though oxygen should not start a fire, it will feed a fire making it burn longer and fiercer.

The doctor can order the blood work needed by many insurance companies to justify coverage of oxygen at home. Results from tests done in the hospital may be admissible if they were done within an acceptable time frame.

Oxygen is a medication and the prescription should be followed accordingly. Flow rates of oxygen should never be increased without the doctor's knowledge and approval. The body may respond to an inappropriate increase in oxygen flow by actually reducing respiratory effort. If the oxygen censor in the brain receives the message that the body is already getting adequate levels, it may send the message to the lungs to slow or cease function. The body cannot identify that the oxygen source is machine made.

Signs will be provided for patients to post in their homes that indicates to all visitors that oxygen is being used. This will discourage smoking in the patient's presence and reduces possible exposure to open flames from lighters.

Patients need to be careful not to trip on oxygen tubing that may have long lengths. If tubing becomes crimped from being caught under furniture, or if it becomes pinched in a door, a high pitched squeal may result. This sound may cause the patient to think that the system is malfunctioning. The patient should turn off the system if they can tolerate being without the oxygen and check for crimped tubing. If the tubing is straightened and the noise persists, the supplier needs to be notified immediately.

Blood Pressure Measurements

Families may obtain products such as electronic blood pressure monitors or thermometers from a medical supplier. These items come with directions for use and often, medical equipment companies will offer technical support by phone.

If the caregiver chooses to monitor the patient's blood pressure himself or is directed to do so by the doctor, the doctor should indicate what values are normal for that patient. The doctor may ask to be called if readings are above or below the patient's normal readings. Regarding the digital blood pressure monitors, the values that are obtained may not be accurate if the machine is not used properly or if the cuff is not placed in the correct position. An abnormal reading should prompt the taker to reapply the cuff and check the results a second time. Blood pressure readings will fluctuate in relation to the patient's activity and medications, so a log that records the patient's blood pressure should also indicate the time of day it was taken, the activity done prior to the reading, and what medications if any where taken by the patient in the hours preceding the reading.

The top number of the blood pressure is the systolic reading and is an indication of how hard the heart is pumping to move the blood out of the heart. This number may increase if the patient is emotionally stressed or has been physically active prior to the reading.

The bottom number of the blood pressure is the diastolic reading and reflects the resistance the blood meets in the blood vessels throughout the body after it has left the heart. The diastolic reading may be increased by any disease of the blood vessels, such as narrowing inside the vessels from plaque buildup, or reduction in elasticity of the blood vessels due to smoking or the aging process. The blood vessels, which provide circulation of blood within the body, can be compared to pipes within the home; their diameter may narrow from frequent disposal of waste that may adhere to the inside of the vessel, or may lose flexibility through long-term use. The doctor can be more specific regarding the patient's disease process and may provide interventions to increase blood flow.

Pulse Taking

The patient's pulse may be monitored by some blood pressure devices, or the family/caregiver can do so manually. The pulse measures how many times the heart beats and is commonly recorded in beats per minute. The doctor will advise if pulse taking is necessary and identify the pulse range that is acceptable for the patient. The most common place to find and count the pulse is in the wrist. This is called the radial pulse. The caregiver should place two fingers just inside the bone on the outer edge of the wrist. This bone can be felt if the patient turns her hand palm up. The caregiver should never use the thumb to assess a patient's pulse because the thumb has its own pulse.

The caregiver can count the beats for 15 seconds and multiply the result by four to get the pulse reading for one minute. If the patient has an irregular pulse, it will need to be felt for an entire 60 seconds because the irregular beats may not always occur in the first 15 seconds. Any irregularity in the rhythm of the beats should be noted and reported to the doctor if it is a new occurrence.

HOME IV THERAPY

This term describes the delivery of medication directly into the patient's body generally intravenously on a continuous or intermittent basis. Home IV therapy also can include enteral care, which is the delivery of medication or nutrition directly into the digestive tract. Some home care agencies provide the care and maintenance for the patient and the equipment themselves; others have contract agencies who provide these services.

Home IV solutions are prepared by a pharmacy that is part of or contracted by the home care agency. The solutions are delivered, sometimes via air mail, from the pharmacy with instruction for storage.

A patient requiring home IV therapy is carefully evaluated prior to acceptance for home care because there are many details involved. There must be adequate electricity and available outlets to run IV administration pumps, proper refrigeration facilities for medication, a safe place for the storage of needles and other supplies, and patient understanding of possible complications from the medication. Manual dexterity to hookup administration tubing is also a factor.

The cost of many IV medications and supplies makes it prohibitive at home unless there is an acceptable environment and teachable patient or caregiver. Insurance companies generally approve home IV therapy if it is administered by a licensed and certified agency, with the doctor's order, and FDA-approved medications. Some insurance companies do not pay for hydration therapy.

Any type of IV or enteral therapy requires a detailed plan for care. There must be a clear understanding of who is involved and exactly what aspect each person or agency is responsible for. Services are coordinated, planned and revised with the doctor's involvement.

Hydration Therapy

One type of care that may be provided is long- or short-term hydration therapy. This is the installation of IV fluids into the patient to establish or maintain adequate fluid balance. The usual method of administration is through an IV catheter that is placed in a patient's vein to deliver the fluids. The catheter may need to be changed every two days or according to the agency's policy. The development of intravenous needles that can be left in longer has made home IV therapy more common. But a patient who needs extended hydration therapy may have underlying concerns that require hospitalization. A patient may need this care for fluid loss from severe or prolonged diarrhea or vomiting which can lead to dehydration.

Nutritional Support

This is available through IV therapy via total parenteral nutrition (TPN). This therapy requires insertion of an intravenous device that is designed to accept a larger volume of fluid, often of greater density than hydration fluids.

The administration site will be accessed more frequently than for hydration, or it may be used for extended periods of time. There is a broad range of intravenous devices available for delivery of TPN, some of which must be placed by a surgeon. These may include a port a cath, PIC catheter or central venous device. The doctor will discuss the advantages of the chosen delivery system and arrange for care of the site as needed, usually by requesting home nursing care. Such IV access sites may also be used for patients that are receiving frequent or very irritating medications on an outpatient basis.

Patients who require TPN are most often referred for home care from a hospital where a delivery system and prescribed formula are established prior to discharge.

Chemotherapy

Administration of chemotherapy at home is another type of IV therapy available. The doctor must administer the first dose of any IV or injected medication in a supervised setting before requesting that the patient receive it at home. This is done to assess the patient's reaction to the medication or treatment, which may need emergency intervention.

Anti-Infectives

Antibiotics may be administered by IV at home to treat infections. They also are only used by patients who have been given the medication before in a supervised setting. The doctor must administer the first dose of IV antibiotics, though it is sometimes considered acceptable to administer a medication in IV form if the patient has tolerated it in oral form.

Home Enteral Therapy

Enteral therapy includes feeding tubes into the nose, stomach or intestine. Administration of liquid nutrition through these tubes is accomplished either with a pump, via gravity or gentle pressure through a feeding syringe. Patients with feeding tubes of any sort are generally unable to provide their own care for the tubes and feeding, so the support system must be assessed carefully. Patients may require enteral therapy when they have difficulty swallowing, or persistent refusal of oral feeding. Frequent episodes of choking while eating or a medical diagnosis that leaves the patient with altered digestion of solid foods may be other reasons to receive enteral therapy.

LABORATORY SERVICES

The increase in home care needs has brought many services to the home that were previously provided in doctors' offices and hospitals. Home blood drawing is one of these services. The doctor must order the type of lab work needed and the frequency. Some labs are able to provide almost immediate home visits for emergency situations.

The addition of home lab service is one of the most valuable tools for medical assessment in the home, allowing the doctor to get a clearer picture of the patient's physiological status and amend care accordingly.

Lab work may be ordered for routine tests weekly, every two weeks or monthly. The need for more frequent lab tests may identify a patient with needs that are better met in a hospital, or who may need to make a doctor visit.

Other tests now available at home include electrocardiogram, fetal monitoring, and portable sonogram. Specific criteria may need to be met when ordering these tests and insurance coverage varies.

The labs are often contracted services of a home care agency and have protocols for distribution of test results. The doctor who ordered the test and the visiting nurse agency are given copies of the test results. Any unusual or abnormal results may be called in to the doctor or nurse from the lab before the written copy is sent.

CONCLUSION

Each of the aforementioned services, from nursing through laboratory work, may be ordered at any time that they become medically necessary. Changes in patient status are evaluated and integrated into the current plan for care, and discussed with the doctor.

Additional services that become necessary during patient care require orders from the doctor to be implemented. A patient has the right to refuse any and all services for home care, but is expected to be available for scheduled visits of accepted services, to inform the nurse or therapist of any changes in his or her status, and to participate in the planned care as able and tolerated.

3

ARRANGING THE ENVIRONMENT

W hen a patient is adjusting to chronic illness or recovering from an acute episode at home, the environment needs to be assessed for safety concerns. Arranging or rearranging each room to meet a patient's specific needs is an issue that a visiting nurse will address. There are general safety measures that apply to all areas of the home, and specific considerations for each room. This chapter summarizes some basic considerations for every patient's general safety.

If it is determined that the environment needs to be rearranged, try to assess the environment from the patient's view. Nostalgic items may provide comfort to the patient and the patient should be consulted before such items are removed. If rearranging the furniture, have the patient move through the room before making the changes permanent.

Consult the patient if possible regarding changes in telephone placement, lighting style, or where bills and important papers are kept. Familiarity with the changes and participation in the arrangements minimizes frustration and confusion for the patient, and maximizes independence.

Reducing clutter can prevent the loss of important or necessary items. Bureaus and other surfaces should be kept clear of unnecessary items. Let the patient be part of the process to reduce clutter. This allows him to maintain some decision-making capabilities, and can help reduce suspicion if items are missing.

REGARDING THEFT AND LOST ITEMS

Because a patient receiving home care services may have several sources of care, including a nurse, therapist, home health aid and others, there is always the potential for personal objects to be missing and the agency caregivers accused.

More often than not, the objects are located later and may even be something that was put away by the patient. If the patient is involved in relocating valuables, he may be able to remember and find the object in question.

Situations where a patient's valuables are missing while care is provided by an agency should be brought to the director's attention immediately. The agency should have an internal policy for resolution. In any situation where virtual strangers are allowed access to a patient's home, this scenario is likely to arise. Be assured that home care agencies are dedicated to providing trustworthy and efficient services and will quickly and effectively address these concerns.

GENERAL SAFETY CONCERNS

Floors

- Floors should be kept dry. Wet tile or other flooring can become very slippery and increase the potential for falls.
- Scatter rugs or runners should be removed or secured to the floor because a corner that lifts even slightly can become a tripping hazard.
- Items that fall to the floor, or that are not usually located on the floor, should be removed. For example, grocery bags, baskets of any sort, shoes or other clothing should not be left on the floor. Piles of newspapers and magazines should be removed not only because of the walking hazard, but for fire safety as well. People become accustomed to their environment and move about without conscious awareness, avoiding familiar obstacles. The addition of debris on the floor provides new obstacles that the patient may not be able to avoid and thus, increases the potential for injury.

Stairs

- Rails on indoor and outdoor stairs should be checked for sturdiness, since they are meant to be used for support when the patient climbs the stairs.
- The installation of a handrail on both sides of the staircase will provide additional support while stair climbing.
- Handrails should be checked for wood splintering. Rough areas can be sanded until smooth.

Doors and Windows

■ Doors and windows should be easy to open and close for an alert patient of average strength.

■ Doors should never lock with a key from the inside; if there is a fire or medical crisis, emergency workers may be delayed in reaching the patient.

■ Window treatments should be kept short to prevent the patient from tripping on long drapes. Hardware should securely hold the blinds or shades in place and cords for blinds should be kept short.

Lighting

■ Lighting should be adequate for the patient to move around in the environment. Lamps that "touch" on or work by sound are available in department, hardware or health product stores.

■ A nightlight that can be left on helps a patient see if he has to get up at night. Many of these devices are light sensitive and turn off automatically during the day.

■ An electrician can install vent lights in the walls to provide a brighter light. These lights are much like those found in hotels and hospitals.

■ Lamps may also be set to turn on and off with a time. This can save a patient a trip down the stairs to turn off a light.

■ Avoid lights that turn on and off with pull strings, especially overhead pulls. The strings can break, or the patient can have trouble accessing the pull. When this happens, the patient may try to climb up to correct the problem, which in turn becomes a safety issue.

Temperature Control

■ Programmable thermostats to raise or lower indoor temperatures help keep the environment comfortable and heating costs down. They also assure that the patient receives adequate heat. They are available in hardware-type stores and include step-by-step directions for use.

Telephones

■ Doorbells and telephones should be checked often for proper function. Intercom devices for the front door can help identify visitors and reduce a patient's rush to get to the door.

■ Phones that have amplified ringers are available through the local phone company, as well as phones that have amplified receivers.

Fire Safety

- If a home has bars or similar safety features on the windows, smoke detectors are critical. In the event of a fire, a patient may need extra time to access the door if window exits are inhibited.

- Carbon monoxide detectors are also an important factor in a safe home environment, especially in older homes whose gas or heating systems may be in disrepair.

- Battery-operated types of both fire and carbon monoxide detectors are available, or an electrician can install them. The advantage of using an electrician is that he or she will place the detectors in the appropriate locations and can wire them directly into the electrical system. This prevents the unit's alarm from ringing when its battery runs low, which reduces unnecessary patient concern and reaction to false alarms. Units that are "hard wired" by an electrician should only alarm if activated by smoke or CO_2. However, they may need to be reset in case of power failure or power surge. Battery-operated alarms need to be checked at least twice a year for function.

- Contact local fire and police departments for information on making the home fire and burglar proof. Many will have a representative visit the home to assess it and make recommendations.

- When possible, fire drills should be planned and practiced.

Pets

- Pets that are already in the patient's home should be kept away from the patient if they pose a tripping hazard. If the patient is emotionally attached to the pet, every effort should be made to keep the pet and have the caregiver supervise its care as needed.

- Pets that become an impediment to patient care because of size, lack of discipline, or involved care should be placed with a person or agency that can provide the necessary care. Patients may be agreeable to this if they can have the pet visit, or if the person caring for the pet is someone they know and trust. Animal control agencies are available to obtain shelter for an unwanted animal. The pet may be placed in temporary shelters or boarded if the patient requires hospitalization. Any arrangements for animals should be noted in the home in case of emergency hospital admission.

- The advantages of keeping a pet are that the patient may be encouraged to participate in its care even when he does not want to participate in his own care.

WHEELCHAIR ACCESS

Patients who have chronic or debilitating disease that confines them to a wheelchair can contact a carpenter or a contractor to help them arrange their environment. Changes may include building ramps in and out of the home for wheelchair access, adding rails at various locations in the home to provide sturdy support for exercise or transferring, and lowering kitchen cabinets so contents can be reached from the wheelchair. Doorways can be widened, doors removed entirely or hinges reversed to change the swing of the door, making it easier to move about.

Working With Contractors

When installing any household device, the manufacturer can be contacted by phone for advice regarding installation and use. The manufacturers' phone numbers should be kept for future reference. However, if you are considering making substantial changes to the environment, you will probably need a contractor. Seek estimates from several contractors first, and ask for their suggestions. Consider exactly what arrangements are most important before making a commitment because structural changes can be costly and time consuming.

Get a written agreement from the contractor detailing exactly what changes are to be made, what they will cost, and a general time frame for completion. If possible, an advocate should oversee the work because the patient may be too fatigued or may have altered thought processes due to disease or medication, and therefore be unable to keep track of the agreement.

Full payment for services should never be made before the work is started. A contractor may ask for a percentage at the start of the job, a second payment after partial completion and the balance when the work is finished. When work includes installation of support devices that may need readjustment shortly after installation, it would not be unusual to hold the last payment until the patient has satisfactorily used the devices for an agreed upon amount of time to assure proper function. A contractor will then be more eager to readjust as needed in order to collect the remaining payment.

Be wary of anyone who comes to the door unsolicited and suggests that the roof needs repair or the chimney needs cleaning. There are many scams like this that target elderly people, who are anxious to prevent any potential problems. So they "hire" the person, but the work never gets done.

Reputable home repair services including plumbers, electricians and carpenters can be located via word of mouth, local union branches, church bulletins, or by contacting the better business bureau. Credentials should be carefully checked before allowing the person into the house and agreeing to their services.

For a patient who owns a home, a general contractor may make scheduled visits to the home and assess repair needs or potential problems. Use of this type of service may help eliminate unnecessary expenses.

SPECIFIC CONSIDERATIONS FOR EACH ROOM

When arranging the patient's environment, focus on the kitchen and bathroom initially. Keep the patient on one floor if stair climbing is difficult. If both rooms are not near each other, but sleeping space is available near a kitchen, this should be the patient's main living area. A commode can be obtained to take care of toileting needs, but kitchen facilities are not generally portable.

Sometimes it may be feasible to have a patient stay in a second-floor bedroom with a bathroom nearby and arrange a small refrigerator and microwave oven on that same floor. This would be most appropriate if the patient has frequent and consistent support to provide groceries and garbage removal. Likewise, use of a commode for toileting would only be an option if it could be emptied on a regular basis. Bed pans are also available through a medical supplier and can be used as an alternative for patients who have difficulty accessing the bathroom.

The Kitchen

Caregivers will likely be responsible for many of the patient's meals. Meal preparation and clean-up should be left to the caregiver as much as possible in order to conserve the patient's energy. However, some patients find it easier to prepare breakfast because it can be a cold meal such as cereal, and their energy level is higher in the morning.

Relinquishing meal preparation is sometimes difficult. Patients often become frustrated when they can no longer provide their own meals, since this is a personal and prideful area of their lives. This is likely the first time a patient will acknowledge the extent of her dependence on others and the limitations of her physical status. To make the transition easier, every effort should be made to allow this patient to participate in meal planning and preparation with supervision as needed.

Preparing and freezing meals that the patient can eat later is an alternative for patients who do not have caregivers available on a daily basis. This is also a way for family members to participate in patient care when time is limited. Be sure that diet considerations are made when preparing foods for the patient, and that they are labeled and dated for easier use.

Foods that are favored by the patient or specific to his culture can be provided by family who are familiar with his tastes. Patients can also enjoy foods specific to the holidays or events that they are unable to attend. This can help reduce feelings of isolation. Soups also freeze well and provide a nutritious meal.

If frozen meals are to be re-heated in a microwave oven, be sure that they are arranged on microwave safe dishes. There are many that can go from the freezer into the microwave.

The temperature of foods and beverages should be checked before giving it to the patient. Microwave ovens may heat food irregularly, leaving the outside steaming hot and the inside cold. More information is presented in the section on diets and nutrition.

Confused or forgetful patients should be kept out of the kitchen as much as possible because of the potential for injury from open flames, gas being left on, broken dishes and glasses, or eating spoiled food.

Stove safety is important. Patients who can use the stove should avoid clothing with wide sleeves, since it may come in contact with flames. A fire extinguisher should be kept in the kitchen for emergencies and the patient and caregiver both instructed in its use. The proper function and contents should be checked frequently and refilled immediately after use.

Delivery services from many stores is available for the homebound patient, or for those who find it easier to have their groceries or meals delivered. Arrangements can be made for weekly delivery of specific pre-arranged items, or called in as needed. Providing groceries and meals to the home is fairly common and many providers have menus and product lists available. A service and/or delivery charge may be added to the cost of the products. The patient or advocate should be aware of such charges and ask for the total of the bill before delivery.

Refrigerator contents should be checked regularly, and any out-dated products should be discarded. The refrigerator should be cleaned and the freezer defrosted to maintain safe and proper function. The contents of the refrigerator should be arranged to help the patient access commonly used items. Food that is in containers with screw caps can be transferred to other storage units for easier access. Large-size products or those in irregular or slippery containers should be avoided.

Cooking and eating areas need to be kept clean to prevent bacteria accumulation. Cutting boards should be checked for mold growth and discarded if noted. Meat preparation and clean-up must be done carefully and thoroughly because the bacteria common to meat can multiply rapidly and may contaminate surrounding counter areas.

Pots and pans should be kept where the patient can reach them, but not behind or above cooking areas. This reduces the chance that the patient will reach past an open flame. Patients may find it easier to leave frequently used pans in the drain after washing.

Adaptive utensils, cups and dishes are available through medical suppliers, pharmacies and mail order catalogues. Some of the best assortment is found at toy stores, such as cups with attachable lids or permanent straws that can reduce spills. Bent utensils or those with straps that hold them on the patient's hand can facilitate transferring the food to the mouth. Dishes with a bottom that can be filled with hot water help keep food warm if meal times are lengthy. However, they should be filled only by a caregiver to prevent injury. Bowls and dishes with suction cups on the bottom can be useful. Bibs, smocks or aprons can be used to protect clothing.

Table top food choppers are a convenient way to mince foods so that they are easier to swallow. Such foods can also be chopped and added to soups or sauces for additional nutrition and fiber as needed. The blades in the chopper are sharp and care should be taken while cleaning them.

Knives and other sharp kitchen implements should be stored at the caregiver's discretion.

Paper or plastic plates and cups can be used if a patient has a communicable disease or frequently throws or drops the dishes. They also reduce the amount of clean-up, which is important if a patient takes care of his own meals.

Coffee pots that deliver coffee directly into an insulated cup are available. This reduces the potential for burns when pouring the coffee. Timers may be used to start any coffee pot or appliance and to turn it off at a set time. This adaptive device can reduce the fire hazard from an appliance that is left on too long.

The Bathroom

The bathroom is an area that can create a large amount of anxiety for the patient. One of the most common fears is that the patient will slip and fall in the bathroom and be unable to get help, or help will arrive to find the patient indisposed.

Most surfaces in the bathroom are tiled and therefore hard, which makes a fall especially hazardous. Water makes these surfaces slippery and increases potential safety hazards. The following is a list of devices and suggestions to make the bathroom more safe. A plumber would be able to obtain and install any of the bathroom adaptive devices, or the medical supply company can provide the equipment and installation services. Bathroom equipment and installation are not generally covered by insurance plans because these items are permanently placed.

Many bathroom adaptive devices seek to reduce the patient's need to bend. The emphasis placed on reducing the need for a patient to bend is important for several reasons. Primarily, when bending down, the patient's blood pressure can alter causing him to become dizzy, or the patient can hit their head on the way back up, lose their balance, or become frustrated if they cannot locate the fallen item.

Tub rails may be used for support. Many patients hold onto towel racks, which are not designed to support a person's weight. Tub rails may be clamped onto the bathtub or installed directly into the walls.

Tub seats allow the patient to sit in the tub without lowering himself to the bottom of the tub. They also help avoid the need to step over the rim of the tub. Tub seat styles vary from basic plastic chairs or benches, to seats that are placed half in the tub and half out allowing the patient to sit down and swing the legs over into the tub. Tub seats are available at medical supply companies and the patient or advocate should carefully assess the patient's current needs, physical strength and capability before purchasing one. If a physical or occupational therapist is visiting the patient, they can suggest an appropriate device.

Sometimes a *basic chair* may be adequate to provide seating in the tub. Those with aluminum frames should be checked for irregular edges that can lacerate skin. If the patient is washing at the sink, a chair in front of the sink for the patient to sit in will make the patient more comfortable and the job less tiresome.

Hand-held shower devices are often used by patients who shower with the aid of a tub seat. These devices allow for complete bathing because of the length of the hose attachment. Some devices may need installation by a plumber, others screw into the existing shower head. Hand-held showers are available from a variety of suppliers including medical supply, hardware and general retail stores. Price comparison may be the deciding factor when choosing a device because they all do primarily the same job.

Non-skid products such as mats and strips should be used, but check them often for lifting or wear. Corners that are not flush with the tub floor can increase the potential for falls. Replace these items often if mildew or residue collects under them.

A *plastic basket* with handles that is filled with the patient's personal hygiene products is very useful. It can be carried into the shower or set down near the sink for easy access. Creating a basket such as this is a thoughtful and useful gift for the patient.

Towels that are buttoned onto the towel rack can help prevent them from slipping off and reduce the patient's need to bend down to retrieve them. Towels such as these are sometimes available in stores, or the patient's own towels can be altered. A thick terry robe can eliminate the need for towels altogether while providing warmth.

Heat lamps that also provide lighting can be installed by an electrician. These systems include fans to reduce steam, but the systems use quite a bit of electricity.

Water temperature should be checked and set at a comfortable level.

Commodes are a helpful and sometimes necessary addition in a patient's home. Every effort should be made to preserve the patient's privacy and self respect when this is the best or only toileting option. Some patients will refuse to use the commode if they are self conscious or embarrassed to have a caregiver clean and empty it. Assure the patient that his or her needs supersede any distaste for this task.

Patients with limited activity tolerance can utilize the commode as a way to conserve energy. The commode can be covered with a sheet or appropriate covering when not in use and the patient assured that when they are stronger, every effort will be made to help them access the bathroom for toilet use.

Portable commodes or bedside commodes can be purchased and used anywhere in the home. This type of portable commode is free-standing and has attached rails. Emptying and cleaning the removable collection bucket must be considered. The contents are disposed of in the bathroom commode and the collection bucket can be sanitized with a bleach solution. Preparations to control odor are available and especially important for a patient who relies on caregivers to empty the contents.

Support devices that fit around the commode in the bathroom can help a patient who has decreased flexibility in the hips that makes sitting down and standing up difficult. Devices that raise the height of the commode seat can be placed directly on the toilet and can be used alone or with the rails.

Flushable wipes for personal hygiene help keep the patient clean, can be used in the bathroom or with a bedside commode and disposed of in the toilet. Wipes should also be kept near the patient who uses a bedside commode for hand washing after commode use.

Liquid soap in a pump container can be used at the sink or in the shower for washing. The dispensers reduce the risk of falling from slipping on bar soap, helps reduce bacteria transfer, and again reduces the patient's need to bend for retrieval.

Electric razors are the best choice for elderly patients especially those with poor vision, reduced manual dexterity, and those taking any kind of blood thinning medication whether prescribed or sold over-the-counter such as aspirin. Disposable razors with blades increase the potential for cuts that may bleed for a longer time if blood thinners are being taken. For those who refuse electric razors, shaving should be done by the caregiver or very closely supervised.

Disposable cups in dispensers are useful for infection control. They also reduce the patient's need to bend to retrieve a fallen cup and prevent glass breakage.

Oral hygiene is important. The toothbrush should be changed every month to reduce infection and provide the best oral care. Patients who prefer it may use mouthwash instead of toothpast on a toothbrush. This is an appropriate choice for patients who have difficulty squeezing toothpaste tubes or expelling toothpaste residue from their mouths. Mouthwash use may be contraindicated because of its alcohol content. A patient who is unreliable and may swallow the mouthwash can have an interaction between the alcohol and his or her prescribed medications. If this is a concern, check with the pharmacist for an appropriate brand of mouthwash that does not contain alcohol. In any case, the patient should always dispense the suggested amount into a separate cup. Never take it directly from the original container. This reduces the chance of overuse and contamination of bottle's contents.

Dentures need routine cleaning, and may need refitting if the patient has had substantial weight loss. Dentures should always be kept in the same container and placed in an accessible location for the patient. Denture loss in the hospital is a common concern, so if a patient is admitted and does not need their dentures for chewing, it would be advisable to keep their dentures at home

Denture containers also need to be kept clean. This can be done with the same products used to clean the dentures. A cleaning tablet can be placed in the container with water and this will reduce bacteria growth. If a container develops a slick film that cannot be removed with denture tablets, replace the container.

In an emergency medical crisis where the patient may need CPR or is seizing, dentures can become an obstacle. Notify the emergency response team if the patient is wearing dentures or is known to have any loose teeth.

Poisonous substances such as cleansers should not be stored in the bathroom where a confused or forgetful patient can access them. Store the solutions where only the person who cleans the house can get to them. At the very least, patients sometimes try to involve themselves in cleaning, and may mistake furniture polish for window cleaner, creating more work. If a patient is insistent about participating in home cleaning, provide them with a spray bottle that is empty or contains water.

A *bell* in the bathroom can provide the patient with independence while performing personal care and access to help if needed. At times it may be appropriate to have a phone installed in the bathroom or provide the patient with a portable phone that they can use to access emergency help if needed.

Water temperatures for bathing should be kept luke warm. Very hot temperatures may cause the blood vessels throughout the body to dilate, which may lower blood pressure and result in dizziness, or may cause burns to the patient's skin.

The Bedroom

One of the most important rooms is the bedroom. Many patients feel comfortable in this room and spend many of their waking hours in it. Visitors may see the patient here and the patient may even choose to have their meals brought to their bedroom. The following is a list of suggestions for enhancing its safety and function.

Adjustable hospital beds, either electric or manual, are available for patient use. Most are rental items that the insurance company may choose to convert to a sale if the patient will need to use it for an extended period of time.

An insurance company will convert a rental to a sale if the monthly rental fees will eventually exceed the purchase price. If a bed sells for $1,000 and rents for $100 per month, the bed is paid for after 10 months. To continue to pay for a rental after those ten months would not be cost-efficient for the insurance company. The disadvantage of such a conversion is that repairs and maintenance on any purchased equipment may become the patient's responsibility. However, there is usually a maintenance and repair contract available for the patient to buy.

Some insurance plans have criteria to determine coverage for an electric bed versus a manual bed. Patients who have breathing trouble that can be improved by raising the head of the bed, or whose medical condition may warrant rapid position change, may qualify for an electric bed. Patients who need a hospital bed for short-term use while recovering from orthopedic surgery may qualify for a manual bed. However, patients who do not have a caregiver available to crank a manual bed to change position may be approved for a manual bed, but have the option of paying the difference between a manual and an electric bed and opt for the latter.

Side rails for a hospital bed must be specifically ordered, and are also available for attachment to many standard beds. An alternative to hospital-style bed rails are the toddler side rails available at most children's stores. This rail can be applied to one side of the bed and the bed placed next to a wall to provide support on the other side, or two rails may be purchased and put on either side of the bed. The advantage to toddler rails is that they are portable and can be used on any size bed. These rails are not as long as hospital bed rails, so determine if two may be needed on one side. They can be placed towards whichever end of the bed the patient needs the most support.

A piece of tape can be placed over the rail-lowering mechanism of most hospital bed rails so that the patient will not be able to access the controls himself. This can help avoid falls or other injuries if a patient needs supervision or assistance getting out of bed. For patients that try to climb over bed rails, position the bed next to a wall to provide access on only one side.

Bumpers can be attached to side rails to cushion them if the patient is restless or pushes an arm or a leg between the rails. Those that fasten by Velcro, snaps or buttons are harder for a patient to remove than those that tie.

Baby monitors in a patient's room can help alert the caregiver to the patient's needs. The monitors can be used for patients who are alert and need intermittent help with some aspects of care. This patient can speak directly into his end of the monitor and make his needs known. For patients who are restless, confused or dependent in their self care, the caregiver can keep her end of the monitor with her regardless of where she is in the home and still hear the activity in the patient's room.

The monitors are especially helpful at night when a patient may not be able to walk to the caregiver's room to ask for assistance. Use of the monitors can increase a patient's feeling of self sufficiency and still allow them easy access to help. And a bell that the patient can ring for assistance can enhance safety and establish an effective bedroom setup.

Preventing pressure sores is important for patients who either spend a lot of time in bed, or do not move around much. There are many products that can be applied to the mattress to provide skin protection by reducing pressure areas. The most common product is the *eggcrate mattress*. This is a foam layer that has eggcrate-like projections. *Plastic air mattresses* with pockets in them that alternately fill with air and deflate are also available. Both provide for relief of pressure to the patient's skin while in bed.

Another alternative is *beds filled with tiny glass beads or sand*. These are available under some circumstances to provide continuous air flow which is not possible with other mattresses. These are specifically ordered for the patient with supporting information from the doctor and nurse explaining why the patient needs this type of bed. Patients who benefit most from this bed are those with wounds to their backside, which are difficult to heal because the patient is unable to stay off the affected area. Medical suppliers set up the bed and provide information regarding its care. Insurance coverage varies for payment of this rental-only item.

Air mattresses are provided by medical supply companies who will apply it to the bed if feasible and demonstrate its care and use. The air mattress must be plugged in to an outlet to function. The appropriate one can be ordered by the visiting nurse on initial or subsequent visits if needed.

Some patients are sent home from the hospital with the eggcrate mattress that was on their bed in the hospital. If it is not offered to the patient at discharge, ask the discharging nurse for it. If the mattress is not soiled, it can then be placed on the patient's bed at home. The eggcrate mattress is a disposable item and will not be re-used by the hospital. The patient and/or insurance company pays for it on the hospital bill. Eggcrate mattresses are popular for patients with skin care needs and now, for the general public as well. They can be purchased at medical supply stores or retail department stores.

Protecting the eggcrate from spills is important because, if it becomes wet or soiled, it must be removed, washed and allowed to dry before re-applying. Heavy soiling may indicate the need for replacement. Methods to protect the bedding and patient from bodily secretions is discussed with the incontinence information.

Eggcrate mattresses may be cut and a piece applied to a patient's chair(s) to provide comfort and reduce pressure on skin when the patient is out of bed. There are a variety of products designed and sized especially for chairs. Medical suppliers can give a patient or caregiver information about each product and help determine which one is most appropriate.

Over-bed tables can be rented or purchased and allow easier set up for meals.

Securing a bag, either plastic or cloth, to the side of the bed can allow the patient easy access to necessary items such as tissues, glasses and magazines. The use of plastic bags should be avoided for patients that reposition themselves in the bed. Plastic bags may be a suffocation hazard for patients that are not fully aware of their environment. Or a *rolling cart* can be stocked with items the patient uses.

Hooks on the back of doors or on walls for robes or frequently used clothes help avoid hangar and closet door use for those with reduced strength or dexterity.

Transfer equipment is available to help the patient move from the bed to a chair or vice versa.

One type is the *Hoyer Lift*, which works by hydraulic pistons. It has a fabric sling that is placed under the patient and then attached by hooks to the lifting device. The lift is pumped by foot or hand, and a rotating arm turns the patient to the desired location. The device then lowers the patient into the chair or bed when the mechanism is released.

Lifts are useful when a patient is either totally dependent with transfers, or the caregiver is not physically able to lift or move the patient by himself. They are ordered by the nurse or therapist with the doctor's approval and they require instruction for the person who will be operating it. Generally, the person being instructed will give a return demonstration to the instructor so proper use is clearly demonstrated. The lift can be a safety hazard if not hooked up or used properly. Lifts also require the proper amount of room for efficient use.

A *transfer board* is another method of assisting the patient from bed to chair. The board is placed between the bed and chair with part of it resting on each. The patient is slid across the board to the chair or if able, slides himself.

The board will work best if the two surfaces between which the patient is transferring are of equal height. If one is higher, it may be difficult to make the transfer against gravity.

The patient should always be encouraged to participate in any activity to the best of his or her ability. Explain to the patient exactly what he is to do so that resistance is minimal. If the patient becomes frightened or confused during a transfer, he could injure himself or the caregiver.

Elevating the foot of the bed can assist circulation. To do this, simply place pillows under the mattress at the foot of the bed. This allows the feet to be elevated without requiring a hospital bed that can do the same thing. Using pillows to raise the feet is also more comfortable and allows an adjustable height to be obtained.

WORKING WITH MEDICAL SUPPLIERS

Many medical suppliers have displays and product information at their retail or warehouse sites. The customer service reps can provide prices and product information as well as alternatives to currently used products if asked. If a patient has a medical condition that may require trying several products before choosing the most effective one, the medical supplier may allow the patient or advocate to look through the product catalogues that the supplier uses when ordering their own stock. These catalogues can sometimes offer a product that the patient had not known was available. If a patient has a colostomy, urostomy, or is diabetic, the supplier may have a specialist available to help the patient with their specific needs.

Mail order catalogues offer a variety of household products that can help keep the patient's bedroom free of clutter. Some mail order companies cater to elderly or disabled people. Local senior citizens groups, social service departments and offices for the aging can provide the names of these companies.

4

MEDICATION

Understanding the medications that are prescribed, and taking the right one at the right time, can make a big difference in maintaining the patient's health. The vital aspects of medication knowledge are: time, dose, frequency, use, action, route, and potential side effects of each medication.

- **Time** refers to the time(s) of day that the medication is to be taken.
- **Dose** refers to the amount of medication to be taken, in pills and in strength.
- **Frequency** refers to the number of times a day the medication is to be taken.
- **Use** refers to why the medication is being given.
- **Action** refers to how the medication works within the body.
- **Route** refers to how the medication will get into the body.
- **Side effects** refers to what the medication may do, aside from its anticipated therapeutic effects.

COMPILE A LIST

To establish an effective medication administration regime, a list of all current prescribed and over-the-counter medications must be made. The medication bottles themselves should be assessed for corresponding information. Things to consider when doing this are: medications that are prescribed by more than one doctor; medications that are prescribed under generic or brand names; and medications with recent change in any part of the administration.

When compiling this list with only the bottles, it is recommended that each doctor be contacted and asked which medications the patient should currently be taking. The doctor can provide the information including the required time, dose and frequency.

Patients discharged from the hospital are sent home with a list of what the doctor orders for medication. This list may not include medications the patient was taking prior to hospitalization. Likewise it may include substitutions for some prior medications. By compiling a written list of all medication in the home and all new written orders, a comparison of medications can be made. Duplicate prescriptions and those for the same medication but with different doses or instruction must be noted and corrected.

The patient or caregiver can review the medications with the doctor or pharmacist. However, a visiting nurse will have the knowledge or resources to identify any discrepancies. In addition, there are books with medication information available for lay people in bookstores. These books are a valuable resource, but may cause the patient undue concern as they tend to list all possible side effects and contraindications. Intervention by a medical advocate is the best solution to establish exactly which medications are to be taken.

Once a master list of current medications is established, take all other prescription bottles and store them away from the current ones. If they are not expired, it is advisable to save them in the event that they are resumed. If this happens, check again that each medication bottle clearly states the dose and name of the medication, and that the dose is the same as the one prescribed.

HELPFUL HINTS

Some medications are filled in generic forms that are generally less expensive. Others may not be available in the prescribed dose and the patient may need to take more than one pill, or half a pill.

It is not advisable to write directions on the pill bottle, such as "take at breakfast," because those orders may change. Nor is it recommended that pills be removed from their original container and stored in other bottles since this may cause confusion if someone other than the patient or primary caregiver is administering the medication.

On the master list, note any other name that the patient may know the medication by, especially if the patient will be the one following the list. General terms such as "the heart pill" may be useful, but make sure that the prescribed name is also listed. Next, write the amount of pills to be taken along with the dose, the number of times per day, the time of day, and any specific administration directions. An example may read as follows: "Lanoxin/Digoxin (yellow heart pill) one .25 mg tablet once a day with breakfast. Take pulse first and if it is below 60, do not take the pill and call the doctor."

Medications that need to be taken at scheduled times of day or with/without food should be clearly instructed by the doctor and supported by the pharmacist's instruction. The prescription bottles should have bold labels with any such instructions.

Medications that cause specific or expected results, such as diuretics causing increased urine output, may require adjustments in administration time to coincide with events, such as doctor visits etc., so that the patient does not experience the side effect at an inconvenient or unmanageable time. The doctor can give the patient or caregiver directions, such as taking half of the dose, skipping a dose altogether or taking it later than the time ordered.

The doctor will clarify specific administration times when prescribing medication. While "bid" calls for doses twice a day, they may be spaced at the patient's liking of morning and night. However, a "q12h" dose must be given every 12 hours, or the second dose taken 12 hours after the first one. Some frequently prescribed medications are available in sustained or time-release forms and the pharmacist or nurse can contact the doctor if this will be more practical.

The nurse can help decipher the frequency and plan with the patient to reduce the number of times per day that the patient must remember to take the pills. Orders for "q4h" (every four hours) might require waking the patient in the night and early in the morning to comply with the schedule. If this is disruptive, the doctor might be able to adjust the order accordingly, but he must be contacted first.

For medications that are ordered "prn" (as needed), the doctor needs to specify what the medication may be used to treat and actions to take if the medication does not relieve the symptoms. This is especially important if treating cardiac conditions. An example would be:

> NTG gr1/150 sl for chest pain, repeat dose q3 min x3 doses, if no relief go to the emergency room or contact MD.

This translates to:

> Place one pill under the tongue, repeat in 3 minutes if the first one does not relieve pain and use a third one three minutes later if the second one does not work. After three doses, if the patient still has chest pains, call the doctor or go to the emergency room for assessment.

If the doctor does not advise what to do if the medication is not effective, ask for a second course of treatment or intervention. Patients and caregivers generally feel more secure knowing that they have a second plan of action so that they do not have to re-contact the doctor. For example:

> Glycerin suppository per rectum if no bowel movement after three days. If suppository does not produce results, repeat one time. If still no results, administer enema.

Doses and strengths of different medications cannot be compared. A diuretic that is 5mg may be just as effective as a different diuretic that is 40mg.

Medication boxes can be pre-filled by the patient or caregiver for up to four different times per day, and up to seven days per week. These boxes, available at drugstores, provide an excellent tool for patients who forget to take their pills, or who are unable to read the pill bottles and could take the wrong medications. Medication boxes are also a solution for patients who are traveling and don't want to take all the bottles with them.

The master list of medication should be posted in the home for all caregivers to reference, and for emergency responders and/or emergency room personnel if necessary. In a medical emergency, the patient may be unable to communicate, or the caregiver may be too overwhelmed to provide accurate information. This list needs to be kept up to date to prevent medication errors. It should include in bold red ink any allergies that the patient has.

Medication Tips

- Store medications as directed, generally out of direct sunlight.
- Always check expiration dates and discard those past the date.

- Dispose of used syringes as directed by the home care nurse. If a nurse is not involved, collect the needles in a container with a lid (heavy plastic jugs from laundry detergent are a good choice), and store it away from children. Also, check with your pharmacist for disposal guidelines. Hospitals often offer services to dispose of used needle/syringe containers.

- The doctor, nurse and pharmacist need to be aware of all documented and possible allergies to medication or foods. This allows for safe and effective prescriptions to be ordered.

- Have the doctor call the prescription in to the pharmacy. This reduces the time spent waiting for a prescription to be filled, and the doctor can clarify any questions regarding the medication administration that the pharmacist may have.

AFTER HOURS

Patients may have questions that occur after customary working hours. When the concern is medical, the general rule of thumb is that a persistent or severe symptom requires medical intervention. The doctor may be called for advice but if a return call is not timely, *go to the emergency room.* Do this by calling 911, or have a family member or friend take you. The emergency room can contact the doctor and will help determine follow-up or treatment needed.

If a medication or treatment is in question, omit it until the doctor can be notified. Better to miss a dose or treatment than take another one that can be potentially harmful, especially if an allergic reaction is a concern.

Regarding medical equipment, many companies have 24-hour on-call services with an operator who is either knowledgeable about the product and can offer trouble-shooting advice, or will relay your question to a company representative. Any agency or supplier that offers 24-hour service does so with the expectation that it will be used by the consumer. Don't feel that you are bothering someone. It's better to be safe than sorry.

THE NURSE'S ROLE REGARDING MEDICATION

The visiting nurse will assess the patient's medication regime as ordered on the referral for home care, or discharge summary sent from the hospital with the patient. If there is not a current medication list available from either source, the nurse will ask the patient or caregiver to see all the bottles of medication that the patient is currently taking, and was taking prior to hospital admission. This includes all medications prescribed by any doctor, those taken over the counter, as well as vitamins.

The nurse will then assess the medication regime for duplication of prescriptions, doses that may not appear appropriate, or medications that conflict. The nurse can also identify any types of medications that are substitutions, which can help prevent overuse of a specific type of medication. Any questions or concerns that the nurse has about the medications will be discussed with the referring doctor, and the information will be relayed to the patient or advocate.

Each nurse may approach the clarification and written instruction in a different way, but the nursing goal is the same: to ensure that the patient or caregiver knows what to take, what it is being taken for, when to take it, the correct dose to take, and any potential side effects or special considerations.

The nursing record that the visiting nurses use as a guideline for their visits will have a list of the patient's current medications. Any changes that occur during the patient's episode of care will be added to the record so that a current list is always available. This is important for caregivers who are not routinely involved in patient care but may be responsible at times for taking the patient to the doctor, reordering medications, or pre-filing a medication box. By keeping an up-to-date master medication list in the home, the nurse can make changes on the list and the nursing record as they occur. That way, even if the caregiver makes only weekly visits to fill a medication box, the master list will be accurate and up to date.

The review and completion of an accurate, up-to-date medication record is one of the most important interventions when a patient arrives home. Patients often assume that they should continue taking the same medications as they did prior to hospitalization, not having been told or not understanding that a medication was stopped or replaced.

One way in which the nurse can be most instrumental in to identify behaviors that the patient exhibits at home that alter the effectiveness or response to a medication. During a hospital stay, diets are prepared by the hospital and are rather exact. This precision may result in the patient needing less of a blood pressure or diabetic medication, for example, while hospitalized. However, on returning home and preparing their own meals, patients may ignore dietary restrictions or follow them more loosely, and their need for the medication may increase or return to pre-hospital doses. The nurse can assess for increases in blood pressure, edema or blood sugar reading, and relay that to the doctor along with the possible cause.

Subsequent nursing visits will include instruction in any and all aspects of each medication. Most agencies have internal classification systems for each medication so that each nurse who visits will provide consistent information.

When a doctor orders injectable medications, the nurse will assess the patient's and caregiver's abilities to learn the injection technique. If the ability to draw up the medication and inject it is consistent and accurate, the patient or caregiver can assume responsibility for administration. There are myriad adaptive devices available to aid independent medication administration, and some of these tools (e.g., magnifiers) may be recommended. Most are available from local pharmacies, but may not be covered by insurance for payment. The nurse will supervise injectable medication administration until independence is obtained and then the patient will be discharged from nursing care if all other instruction regarding disease process and self care is attained.

Diabetic patients can be instructed in the use of blood glucose monitoring machines. Generally, this instruction takes place at the same time as instruction in administering insulin injections.

For diabetic patients, caregiver involvement is especially helpful because of the amount of knowledge that needs to be transferred. In addition to injection administration and instruction, patients may need to learn how to adjust insulin doses according to the results of blood glucose testing. Written instructions in all aspects of injection technique and glucose testing, along with specific and clearly stated orders for insulin adjustments if prescribed, will be provided by the nurse upon doctor's order receipt.

In the event that the patient or caregiver is unable to perform some or all of the injection procedure, the nursing interventions will be modified. Some patients cannot see well enough to draw up the correct dose of medication, but are able to administer it correctly. In this event, the nurse may be able to visit on a modified basis to pre-fill syringes with the medication, and the patient will be responsible for administering it. Some insurance companies do not pay for nursing visits to pre-fill syringes in which case the patient may choose to pay privately for this service. Such visits by the nurse to pre-fill syringes should also include an assessment of the patient's blood pressure, heartbeat and general physical status with attention to body functions that relate to the patient's diagnosis. Any changes in the patient's status or in the medication regime may signify a need for the patient to resume nursing care. In the event that a competent caregiver is unavailable for a period of time (taking vacation or undergoing medical treatment herself), the nurse may visit for that period of time to administer the medication.

In some cases, the patient will never be capable of preparing and administering an injectable medication and no caregiver is identified to assist. This scenario is most common with insulin-dependent diabetic patients. Common effects of diabetes include visual disturbances and/or loss of sensation in the hands, which decreases manual dexterity and renders the patient incapable of self injecting. Another common problem is the alteration of thought processes, leaving the patient unable to remember to take the medication. In this event, the nurse will contact the doctor and establish a plan for patient care that may include daily or twice-a-day administration of medication according to insurance allowances. The insurance company will compare the cost of frequent home nursing visits to the cost incurred by the patient being placed in a hospital or institution.

In the case of a patient who is independent in all aspects of care except for oral medication administration, every effort will be made to locate and teach a family member or friend how to pre-fill a medication box. The same effort is made with injectable medication, but the caregiver needs to have a greater availability for both instruction and care.

For medication with other administration routes, such as eye drops or suppositories, the patient may need fewer skills. For instance, with a suppository, the patient does not need extremely precise visual skills to administer it safely and efficiently. Manual dexterity is a more important factor.

Eye drops can be somewhat more confusing because some are given to one eye, some to the other, and/or some to both. Most eye drop bottles are tiny and the writing on them is small. If the patient always takes the drops while in the same location of the house or room, the bottles for the right eye can be placed to the patient's right and those for the left eye to his left. If this plan is used, a caregiver must periodically check that the bottles' locations are correct.

Medication that is given through a feeding tube requires nurse instruction to the caregiver for proper administration technique. The nurse can also help determine which medications may be crushed for easier administration, or which are available in liquid form. The nurse may need to check first with the pharmacy to help determine which medications are still effective after crushing; extended release medications will lose their potency and their expected results will be reduced if crushed. If medications need to be crushed, commercial pill crushers can be purchased to make this easier and more effective, or a mortar and pestle can be used.

THE PHARMACIST

The pharmacy and pharmacist are valuable tools in rendering care to a patient at home. For patients with limited medical resources, a pharmacist who knows the medication regime can answer questions about the actions and possible side effects if the doctor is not available. The visiting nurse may use the pharmacist for information on medications that are new or experimental, or to clarify the best times for administration if the patient is taking a large number of prescriptions. Further, the pharmacist can identify over-the-counter medications that are compatible with the patient's prescribed regime if, for instance, a doctor orders a patient to take cold or cough medication without ordering a specific brand. Some preparations are low in salt or sugar, or some may interact negatively with prescribed drugs.

The following are some services that a pharmacist may provide when asked, and can be a great benefit to a patient. When looking for a new pharmacy, these services should be considered. It is always possible to transfer prescriptions to a new pharmacy if it offers better services.

- Twenty-four hour availability to call in prescriptions or obtain refills.
- Home delivery service. A pharmacy can also deliver any of the products available in the store when delivering a prescription. A patient may request a specific product, or ask the pharmacist what he or she may recommend to meet a specific need, such as a cough or a cold, or soft supplies for incontinence, etc.
- Pre-cut the medications if the dose order requires a partial tablet. Pill cutters are also available for purchase.
- Let the patient know if any of his current medications should be taken at a specific time in relation to food or other medications.
- Provide written information—although it's usually routinely offered—or a verbal explanation of the medication's actions, use, dose and potential side effects.
- Inform the patient as to what types of packaging are available to make the medication easier for the patient to access, or harder if children are in the home.

5

BASIC ASPECTS OF GOOD CARE

INFECTION CONTROL

Prevention is one of the single-most controllable aspects of infection control. Care should be taken by both the personal caregiver and the patient before and after any patient contact in order to prevent and control contamination. This helps cut down on the transfer of bacteria and viruses. Infection control is necessary regardless of the patient's diagnosis. It is not dependent on a diagnosed infection. Bacteria common to one person may cause an infection in another person whose immune system is compromised because of medication, age or the presence of open skin that allows bacteria to enter. The following is a list of infection control techniques that are appropriate for any and all persons who are ill or who are caring for a patient in the home.

Handwashing

Wash hands before and after any contact with the patient and/or their body fluids. Bacteriostatic liquid soap in a dispenser is the easiest and most appropriate choice of hand cleansers because bar soap may retain bacteria. If bar soap is used, hold the bar under hot running water to clean it before use.

Hands should be washed from the cleanest area to the dirtiest; that means from the wrist to the fingers. Hold hands with the fingers facing down into the sink so the water will wash over the hand in that direction. Clean between the fingers with soap and water, and twist any rings on the fingers so the soap and water go under the ring and onto the skin.

Dry hands on a paper or other disposable towel. Cloth towels may harbor bacteria and re-contaminate hands. This may seem like a basic process, but it is a first important step in infection prevention.

Hand washing is especially important when there is contact with body fluids. It will help prevent contamination of the caregiver as well as the patient. If body fluid waste is being handled on a regular basis, as with an incontinent patient or for wound care, disposable gloves are advisable. Many types are available at local pharmacies. It is also wise for a caregiver who has to apply ointment to a patient's skin to use gloves, as the medication in the ointment may be absorbed into the caregiver's skin.

For a personal caregiver with sensitive skin, frequent handwashing and glove use may aggravate hands. Using hand lotion or powder-free disposable gloves may help.

Laundry

Linens and other washable materials that come in contact with the patient's body fluids should be washed separately from the rest of the household's. Heavily soiled items may need to be soaked. This can be done with household bleaching products or the addition of baking soda to the laundry. When soaking materials in bleach, be sure they are rinsed well before washing to prevent chemical injury to the patient's skin.

Perspiration is considered a body fluid and may become contaminated from medications or infections that are transferred out of the patient as waste via sweat glands. The pharmacist or doctor should provide this information if pertinent. Other body fluids that come into contact with clothing and linens include feces, urine, oral secretions, and drainage from open wounds on the patient's body. For this reason, pillowcases must also be changed frequently and washed with soiled linen. It is better to err on the side of caution, because the introduction of harmful bacteria is often very preventable through use of hygienic techniques.

Garbage Disposal

Garbage from the patient should always be double bagged before disposal. Such items that come into contact with body fluids may include tissues, straws, disposable plates, cups and napkins, disposable gloves, dressings, and incontinence products. An easy way to incorporate this action is to place double bags in all of the patient's garbage cans. Check bags for holes prior to use to prevent accidental dumping of their contents. Double bagging is used to prevent contamination of those who handle the garbage both inside the home and out.

There is no need to label the bags as medical waste unless the patient is receiving treatment at home with hazardous chemicals or syringes. If this is the case, the person or agency providing the treatment will provide either specific disposal guidelines or will remove the waste itself to ensure proper disposal.

Gloves

Heavyweight reusable kitchen gloves may be used in some cases instead of disposable gloves. They are cost effective, especially in the case of incontinence care, and helpful with handling soiled linens and clothing. They would not be an appropriate choice, however, for wound care because of the potential for contamination.

If using utility or kitchen gloves, the caregiver needs to protect her own skin because bacteria may grow inside the gloves. Cotton gloves may be worn inside them to prevent contact with bacteria, but the cotton gloves must then be washed regularly as well.

Masks

Caregivers who have upper respiratory infections and must continue to provide patient care can use masks to help prevent spreading their infection to the patient. The mask covers the nose and mouth and reduces the spread of bacteria and viruses found in respiratory droplets.

A mask is also good for patients who have respiratory infections that produce frequent or large amounts of discharge when coughing or sneezing. This is particularly important if the caregiver himself or herself is immunosuppressed, whether the result of disease or cancer treatments.

Sterilization of Eating Utensils

Dishes and cutlery can be washed with usual dish detergent, or placed in a dishwasher if available. The high heat and repeated water flow of a dishwasher can help prevent bacteria re-growth.

NUTRITION AND HYDRATION

The nutritional needs of a patient vary with age, disease process and medication regime. As a person ages, the ability to chew, swallow and digest may be affected. Chewing can be limited because of disease, poor mouth care, ill-fitting dentures, tooth loss or an alteration in neurological or muscular coordination. Swallowing can be difficult due to medications or loss of muscle coordination due to the disease process, such as from stroke. The digestion of foods may be altered by the disease process, medication or the body's inability to breakdown complex foods.

Oral Hygiene

Mouth care is the first important step towards good nutrition. Mouth care should always be performed while the patient is sitting upright to prevent choking on fluids. If the patient is unable to be positioned upright, the caregiver needs to turn the patient's head to the side to facilitate drainage of cleaning liquids and sputum. To perform mouth care for a dependent patient, first wrap and secure a soft, small gauze pad to a toothbrush or tongue depressor. Then dip the end in lemon-glycerin solution, peroxide or baking soda and water, or mouthwash. Use this swab to gently wipe out a patients mouth. Commercially prepared lemon-glycerin swabs are available for purchase. If a patient has sores in his mouth, avoid solutions that contain alcohol because they can be irritating and painful.

This type of mouth care cannot be used for patients who bite down on the swab because the wrap may dislodge and become a choking hazard. Patients that have difficulty swallowing should also not have any liquids introduced into their mouth. For these patients, a soft tooth brush may be used, especially if they have their own teeth.

Any bleeding, blisters or sores on the gums, lips or lining of the mouth should be relayed to the doctor. A variety of medications to treat this condition are available both over the counter and by prescription. Vaseline or other oil-based lip preparations can be applied to soothe dry lips. However, they must be avoided if the patient receives oxygen at home because the petroleum base is potentially flammable. Instead, a water-based product such as KY Jelly may be substituted.

Nutritional Concerns

Generally, patients should eat and drink in a sitting position unless contraindicated by their medical condition. Small amounts of food should be offered by fork or spoon, and frequent rest periods allowed. Small and frequent meals are often easier for the patient to tolerate since it reduces the energy needed for chewing, swallowing and digestion. Never force a patient to eat by putting food into their mouth. And always allow ample time for swallowing.

A healthy diet should consist of a balance between fat, protein, fruits/vegetables and carbohydrates. A sample of foods to offer might include toast, applesauce, yogurt, fruit, sweet potatoes, minced meats, cottage or other soft cheeses and pureed vegetables. Eggs and beans provide a good source of protein that can be served in a small portion and easily prepared with vegetables or cheese for a balanced meal. They can also be easily pureed and added to soups.

Diet restrictions, if any, should be discussed with the doctor and a copy of the diet obtained for the caregiver and visiting nurse. Bookstores, libraries and disease-specific groups (such as the American Heart Association) can also provide diet information.

There are many foods that are thought to prevent disease or ease symptoms. Registered dietitians can be consulted for nutritional counseling and are sometimes available by consult through home care agencies.

Adequate nutrition is important to maintain health and provide energy. Every effort must be made to provide the patient with foods that he will eat and are easily digestible. The patient's food preferences should be taken into consideration when preparing or planning meals. If many caregivers are involved in meal preparation, this can be documented so that everyone has the information.

If the patient has a preference for a food or food group that is not included in the prescribed diet, the doctor or dietitian may offer substitutes or allow small infrequent use. In this case, be sure that specific amounts of that food, and the frequency with which it can be served, are clearly spelled out because judgment of portion size and frequency may vary from person to person.

Sometimes, specific foods or food groups are either encouraged to enhance the patient's medical status, or limited because they interfere with the patient's medical regime. For example, adding fruits and vegetables to the diet can provide roughage to aid bowel elimination, but may be contraindicated for certain gastrointestinal diseases. Foods rich in protein may hasten wound healing, but quantities may be restricted if some diseases such as kidney failure are present.

Some foods that may be limited are high-sugar foods and carbohydrates for those with diabetes, and high-sodium foods for those with hypertension. Restrictions of protein, cholesterol and fat may also be made, depending on the diagnosis and treatment regime. Sores in the mouth can become more irritated with the use of spicy or acidic foods such as citrus derivatives, vinegar and pepper, and these types of foods would be restricted.

When possible, fresh foods should be used because they are most rich in nutrients. For nutritionally conscious patients or those whose nutrition is poor, vegetables can be steamed and the water from steaming used to boil pastas or used in soups. Vegetables can be pureed and added to soup stocks, both to thicken them and increase their nutritional value. Fruit nectar may be substituted for fruit juice to provide thicker liquids and less acidity.

Pasta products that are made with vegetables in the flour itself are available at grocery or food specialty stores. These can add some nutrients to the patient's diet. Small pasta products such as pastina can be mixed with pureed meats, vegetables or cheese to add carbohydrates.

Pre-packaged foods can be used, but frozen, processed or canned foods may be high in sodium. Reduce the use of these products or use the lower-sodium variety. Rinse canned vegetables in tap water and cook them in water to reduce their salt content.

Jars of baby food may add variety and ease to food choices. The small size allows for less waste and the consistency is especially good for those with difficulty swallowing.

Shakes can be made from yogurt, fruit and sherbet or fruit juices. This is another way to provide nutrient-dense products for a patient with limited energy or ability to eat.

Gelatin products can be made, cooled slightly and then drank before they set completely. The patient will receive the protein available from the gelatin without having to chew. Another source of protein is fortified milk, which is available in low-fat forms.

Any specific increase or use of vitamin and mineral supplements should be checked with the doctor.

It is important to note a patient's tolerance when new foods are introduced. Assess the patient for rashes, stomach upset or change in bowel movements. Products that do not agree with the patient should be noted and avoided. Patients who are not able to communicate discomfort may indicate it by drawing up the knees towards the abdomen, grimacing when the food is offered, or by a change in bowel elimination frequency or consistency.

Food Labels

Labels on food products provide accurate nutritional information and can assist the caregiver in planning meals. Food labeling laws have become stricter regarding broad terms such as sugar free or low fat. A free brochure that details these guidelines is available through the Food and Drug Administration (1-800-532-4440).

Food labels allow people to monitor their diets more effectively, especially when given restrictions. In the event that the doctor orders a low fat, low sugar or low salt diet, ask that the doctor specify the number of grams allowed so that controlled intake is more possible. Any food product that comes packaged without a nutritional breakdown should be avoided, or its use limited.

Fluids

Patients with unrestricted fluid intake should drink six to eight 8-ounce glasses of fluids per day. The patient's fluid intake may be limited by the doctor because of disease process or the patient's tolerance. Or the patient may be encouraged to increase his fluids. In either case, the doctor will order a specific number of ounces or ml/cc (milliliters or cubic centimeters) to be taken in during a 24-hour period.

Any specific amounts of fluids that the doctor orders should be communicated to all caregivers. It is helpful to have a flow chart established where the caregiver can write down exactly how much the patient has had to drink while under her care. This helps eliminate potential over- or under-hydration that can lead to alterations in fluid and electrolyte balances causing a multitude of problems within the patient's body.

In the event that the doctor's fluid restrictions are exceeded, the doctor should be notified. The doctor may suggest that the patient be monitored for signs of fluid overload specific to the patient and his disease process, or the doctor may order correction by medication. If a gross excess occurs, the doctor may order lab work to help determine the effects on the patient.

Clear fluids offer the best hydration value, but fruit or vegetable juice may be choices for nutritional supplements. Coffee and tea may be used if fluids are unrestricted, but caffeine-free varieties are the best due to caffeine's effects on the body, such as an increase in heart rate or palpitations. Sports drinks are high in electrolytes and should not be used unless the doctor orders them because the concentration may be too high for the patient to tolerate.

If swallowing is difficult for the patient, thickeners for fluids can be recommended by the doctor. Some patients may find it easier to swallow through a straw or take sips of water prior to eating to moisten the throat and ease swallowing.

Dehydration can occur if the patient does not receive an adequate amount of fluids either by mouth or through feeding tubes. Dehydration is also a problem with prolonged vomiting or diarrhea, and with hot weather and high temperatures. Signs of dehydration include but are not limited to: confusion, dry mouth or lips, dry skin, generalized weakness, rapid heart rate and lowered blood pressure. These symptoms are broad and can be attributed to many other sources such as the disease process or use of certain medications. Lab work can reveal other clues to the cause of these symptoms.

Liquid nutritional supplements are available in cans and can provide calories, vitamins and minerals. Some patients may find that the supplements alter bowels, are not to their taste, or may be expensive. If the doctor recommends a supplement and the patient finds it difficult to use, ask the doctor to recommend a replacement.

Elimination

If stools are loose, diet adjustments to include bananas, rice, applesauce, toast and cheese may help. Apple sauce contains pectin that helps firm bowel movements but is not contained in apple juice. Rice may be boiled in water and the remaining liquid cooled and then consumed either orally or through a feeding tube to reduce diarrhea. Commercial diarrhea preparations should only be used with the doctor's permission because they may actually make the body re-absorb the bacteria or virus causing the loose stool, making the patient sicker.

Constipation may be relieved with the addition of bran or fiber in the diet, along with adequate fluid intake. Over-the-counter remedies for constipation may be suggested by the doctor and taken according to package information. Some of these medications work best in combination, and several may need to be tried before an efficient regime is established. There are also herbal teas available to reduce constipation but the patient should be frequently evaluated for side effects of the other contents of the tea that can cause stomach upset or rash.

RESPIRATORY HEALTH

Patients who are confined to bed or have limited mobility can't participate in normal activities such as walking up stairs, cleaning and gardening, and their respiratory health can suffer as a result. It's important for these patients to cough and perform deep breathing exercises to help expand their lungs.

Air intake causes the lung to expand, which allows optimal oxygen absorption. Lack of fresh air flow can facilitate the growth of bacteria because lungs at their furthest point can be dark, warm and moist. This bacterial growth can get trapped in the natural mucous of the lung and respiratory infection such as pneumonia can then occur.

Encourage the patient to take three to four deep breaths in through the nose and out through the mouth. Have them perform this exercise four times a day to enhance gas exchange in the lungs. If the patient becomes short of breath or dizzy during the exercises, stop, have them rest and call the doctor if the symptoms are persistent or severe.

6

SKIN CARE

It is important for all patients, regardless of their activity and dependence levels, to keep their skin clean and dry. Patients should be washed or bathe themselves on a daily basis using water and non-drying soap. Any skin care product that contains perfume can dry the skin because of the alcohol in the perfume. Glycerin or lotion-based soaps provide added moisture while cleaning. There are also a wide variety of ointments and lotions available for application after washing. Oils and lotions that contain fruit, nut or other natural derivatives may turn rancid after exposure to light and warmth. To avoid this, read the label for such a warning and if in doubt, contact the manufacturer for advice.

SKIN BREAKDOWN

Skin breakdown is one of the biggest concerns for a home care patient. A patient with any disease process or complication that reduces their ability and/or desire to move about or change position is at increased risk for skin breakdown. Patients who spend frequent or extended periods of time alone may be less motivated to be active. Both situations predispose a patient to skin breakdown from the increased pressure and reduced circulation that occur when activity is limited. Areas that may be affected are not only the buttocks, but also posterior thighs, elbows, heels and along the spine. Understanding how and why the skin deteriorates can lead to a better understanding of preventive measures.

- Contact with irritating liquids such as urine or feces can cause the skin to breakdown.
- Pressure from the bones under the skin, and a lack of cushioning externally, increases the potential for pressure sores to develop.

■ Shearing of the skin, caused when the skin is pulled in one direction and the underlying bone does not move with it, causes skin to break down.

The following skin care suggestions apply to all causes of skin breakdown and are basic principles of good skin care.

Cushioning

The skin of an elderly patient is often fragile under the best of situations due to poor fluid intake, slowed cell regeneration and loss of elasticity due to age. It is important to provide cushions or special mattresses for the patient to rest upon. Such cushions reduce the external pressure on the skin by providing a soft barrier between the patient's bones and the surface they are sitting or laying upon.

If commercial mattress pads are unavailable or costly, placing a thick terry cloth towel either directly under the patient, or beneath the sheet to provide some cushioning. An added advantage of a towel is the ease of washing it when it becomes soiled.

Imagine what happens to a paper towel if it is placed between a heavy pot or other weighty, firm object and a hard counter top. If the pot is slid across the counter with or without added downward pressure, the paper towel will eventually fray from the pressure exerted on both sides. If water is added to the paper towel, the tearing will happen faster and may be more extreme. This is what happens to the skin, especially with the addition of body fluids such as perspiration or urine that may be irritating even without contributing pressure or friction.

Position Changes

Patients that are able to walk or transfer to a chair should be encouraged to do so every one to two hours. This changes the pressure on the skin, as well as increases the blood circulation. If a patient is confined to bed because of long-term alterations in activity tolerance, the caregiver should turn and reposition the patient every hour or as directed by the nurse or doctor. This is done by placing the patient on one side of her body, then on her back and then on the other side. Positions that cannot be tolerated because of discomfort or medical contraindications should be avoided. The patient's position may be dictated by tolerance. If a patient has an open skin area, even 15 minutes off of the affected area can increase circulation and aid healing.

Levels of discomfort may be assessed to determine if the patient cannot tolerate a certain position, or is simply resisting the change. Charts may be used to record what position a patient was in and for how long if several caregivers are involved. Similarly, schedules can be made to assure that changes occur.

Moving a Dependent Patient

To prevent a shearing-type of skin injury, a draw or pull sheet can be used. This can be made by taking a flat sheet and folding it in half then placing it under the patient, leaving room on either side to grab a handful of the sheet. If two people are available, one person stands on one side of the patient and the other stands on the other side. Each person holds the top and bottom corners of the sheet on their side. At the same time, both people pull the sheet toward the top of the bed taking the patient along with it. This technique allows for equal distribution of the patient's weight and the sheet is pulled, not the patient.

If one person is using a pull sheet, he can stand at the head of the bed, behind the frame, and hold the top of the sheet that is under the patient's shoulders. By using a pull sheet, the sheet moves the patient, reducing friction as well as the amount of energy the caregiver must use.

When trying to move a dependent patient up in bed without a pull sheet, it is not uncommon to have the patient move up only slightly, and quickly slide back down. This is because the patient's skin is really all that moves, not the patient's body frame. The bones underneath the patient then rub the skin from the inside and the patient's skin rubs the sheet on the outside. If done frequently and/or forcefully, a skin sore can develop. If a patient is alert and physically able, she can be instructed to bend her knees and dig her heels into the bed to push herself up towards the head of the bed.

A pull sheet can also be used to help turn the patient on her side. First, use the pull sheet to move the patient closer to the side that they are turning off of. Then, with the caregiver's hands holding the sheet close to the patient's body, pull the sheet and roll her on the side she is to be positioned on.

To put a clean pull sheet on the patient's bed, roll the patient on his side and drape the old pull sheet over his hip, or if heavily soiled, roll it up and push it deep under his side. Take a new pull sheet and place it so that half is laying flat on the bed where the old one was; then roll the other half up tightly. Push the rolled pull sheet under the soiled one or under the patient with the flat half smoothed out on the bedside behind the patient. When the patient is rolled onto his other side, the caregiver can reach under the patient and remove the soiled sheet, then unroll the clean pull sheet that is next to the patient's skin. It may take a few attempts before the caregiver is able to judge how much of the pull sheet needs to be rolled and how much left flat. The nurse can demonstrate this technique during a visit.

Position changes should be done slowly and carefully because sudden changes can alter the patient's comfort and blood pressure. Patients that are getting out of bed should reposition themselves from lying to sitting at the edge of the bed for a few minutes first, to allow their blood pressure to adjust to the position change. The patient should only stand if no dizziness exists.

Pillows, rolled blankets or towels can be placed behind the patient to help maintain position. Folded towels should be placed between the patient's knees or ankles to help maintain body alignment, to provide comfort, and to reduce friction between the bones that can lead to skin breakdown.

The toes of a long cotton sock can be cut off and the remaining length pulled up over a patient's arm to provide a cushion for elbows, helping prevent pressure and shearing of skin at that site.

Special considerations need to be made for patients with contractures (permanent muscle tightening). These muscles lose the ability to move healthy blood to and through them, which naturally occurs when muscles contract and relax, squeezing surrounding blood vessels and enhancing circulation. Nourishment and oxygen are provided by blood flow and these help maintain healthy tissue. Additionally, contracted muscles often result in two body parts being in constant contact. For instance, contractures in the lower leg can cause the leg to be drawn up so that the calf and posterior thigh meet, and contractures in the fingers and hands can cause fists to remain clenched. Air flow is reduced and this creates a dark, warm, moist environment– the breeding ground for bacteria.

Special consideration for the hand include keeping fingernails short and even to prevent laceration of the palm. Gauze pads or pieces of cloth can be inserted between the fingers to absorb moisture. Rolled or folded hand towels can be placed in any other area to prevent bones from rubbing together. A thorough check of the patient's skin should be made twice a day to assess for changes.

Hot Spots

Areas of skin that are closed but appear soft, discolored, hot or tender may indicate that the underlying tissue is not receiving adequate blood supply. This may eventually lead to open sores. These areas need pressure relief provided by mattress pads, position change and basic skin care.

Heating pads must be used carefully and according to the manufacturer's direction. It is not uncommon for a patient to get a burn from misuse. Several types of heating pads can turn on and off in cycles, or can be used with moisture to increase heat distribution and prevent burning.

Other areas that may become a problem are ear lobes that are pressed between the patient's head and the pillowcase, the skin between the toes and fingers, and any area where two bones rub together such as the inner knees. A rolled hand towel can be secures with tape and placed in the patient's hands to provide a barrier between fingers and the palm. Soft gauze pads can be placed between toes to reduce friction and absorb moisture.

Soft materials such as lambskin can be used to pad chairs and reduce pressure. Lambskin is available from commercial stores or medical suppliers and can be cut into pieces.

Treatment

Any changes in the skin or suspected breakdown should be made known to the doctor. A treatment plan can be implemented and the visiting nurse referred for instruction or care as needed.

In the event that a patient develops an open sore, the nurse who is referred will assess the wound for size, location, drainage, possible cause and prevention of further breakdown. It is not uncommon for the doctor to order specific wound care after a nursing assessment.

When possible, the nurse will instruct caregivers in the wound care procedure, assess their ability to perform the care correctly, and make return visits to assess the patient's healing and alter the plan as needed. If a caregiver is unwilling, unable or unavailable, the doctor can order that wound care be performed by the nurse. This may necessitate daily or twice-daily care. When able, the nurse and doctor will chose a treatment that is effective and can be done less frequently. Since insurance plans tend to limit the frequency of nursing visits, such involved home care may require ongoing justification of the planned visits with notations about the continued lack of patient's ability or caregiver involvement.

The type of wound care can range from simple dressings to complicated step-by-step regimes. A variety of medications for irrigation or installation into the wound bed are available. The regime is determined by the type of wound and location, as well as the patient's response to treatment. The nurse will instruct the patient or caregiver in the storage and care of products used for wound care. Home health aids are generally prohibited by practice standards from performing all wound care. As a rule, all medications and ointments should be stored out of direct sunlight and away from extreme temperatures.

DRAINAGE

Any drainage that is crusted should be loosened before removal, regardless of location. Pulling or forcefully wiping drainage that has adhered to the patient's skin can damage the underlying tissue and remove growth of new tissue if on a wound.

Any drainage that is green or yellow in color, foul smelling, bloody, purulent (contains pus) should be brought to the doctor's attention. These are potential signs of infection and may need immediate intervention. Likewise any skin that is red, hot, tender or swollen, or any fever or chills can indicate an infectious process that is not yet visible. The doctor may advise specific fever-reducing methods or medication, or he may advise to let the fever take its course. However, check with the pharmacist before administering any over-the-counter medications for fever reduction, especially if they contain aspirin. Aspirin is a known blood thinner and can also irritate the stomach. The pharmacist may recommend an alternative or she may check with the doctor for an appropriate medication.

CIRCULATION

Elderly patients commonly have reduced circulation, either due to their medical diagnosis or as the general results of aging. If circulation problems are diagnosed, the doctor may offer specific medications or treatments to correct or reduce complications. Using skin lotion provides moisture replacement and a barrier from friction, and the application of the lotion allows for massage of the affected area which increases blood flow.

Ointments and other skin barrier preparations should only be used on intact skin. The doctor, pharmacist or visiting nurse can suggest specific brands, but several may need to be tried before determining the most effective product. Some ointments are designed to provide a water-resistant barrier for the skin but may be difficult to wipe off. Others may change their consistency and effectiveness if they come in contact with body fluids. For those that contain vitamins or medications that are absorbed by the body, check with the doctor or pharmacist before applying to prevent any interactions with the patient's medication regime. As mentioned previously, some medications that come in ointment form can be absorbed by the person who is applying it; the use of gloves will eliminate this potential problem.

Avoid using tight shoes and slippers because they reduce the circulation in the feet and can cause skin irritation from pressure or friction. Loose cotton socks are the best type of footwear because they allow for air flow and will not constrict blood vessels if they are loose enough. The rule is, any footwear that leaves an indentation is too tight.

Reduced circulation to the legs or feet may occur either because of a medically diagnosed condition, or naturally because blood vessels lose elasticity as a person ages. Altered circulation to the legs or feet can result in swelling (edema). The effects of edema can lead to skin breakdown due to the stretching of the skin and the reduction in healthy blood flow that normally removes waste from cells. The accumulation of waste leads to less room in the cells for oxygen and nutrients, which is required for optimal function. Cells that are not properly supplied with these elements die. Accumulation of dead cells under the skin increases the potential for skin breakdown externally, much as bruised areas in a piece of fruit eventually make the fruit's skin wither.

If swelling of the legs or feet is noted, the doctor needs to be notified so a treatment plan can be developed. The plan may first be to raise the feet to help gravity return the blood to the heart and encourage the return of healthy blood to the area. The use of a reclining chair helps to keep the feet in an elevated position. Sodium in the diet may also be restricted because an increase in sodium may increase fluid retention.

The doctor may also advise the use of diuretics, which are medications that increase the body's ability to excrete excess fluids through urine output. The doctor, nurse or pharmacist will advise on the use and potential side effects of these and any other medications.

Swelling of the legs and feet may also be caused by heart disease that can render the heart unable to efficiently pump the blood out of the heart, or to facilitate blood flow back to the heart. Kidney disease may also alter the body's ability to remove excess fluids, and the body may store the remainder in the feet or legs. There are also diseases of the cell function that reduce the body's ability to transfer waste out of the cells and vital elements in. The doctor should explain the specific disease process and how it affects swelling to the patient and caregiver so they are of aware of complications and can do what is necessary to prevent them.

The nurse assesses swelling by how the skin responds to pressure (pitting). The nurse may weigh the patient because increased weight may signify increased water retention. Or the nurse may measure specific points on the leg or foot to assess for increased size that would signify swelling.

The patient or caregiver will be instructed in ways to reduce or prevent swelling, as well as how to assess for changes in swelling. The doctor may order that the patient use support hose, which can be obtained from medical suppliers. These require measurement of the patient's legs for proper fit. The nurse or advocate from the medical supplier can help with these measurements.

FOOT CARE

Foot care is important for all patients, especially those with impaired circulation to the feet either as a primary diagnosis or as a side effect of a disease process such as diabetes. The feet should be washed daily and inspected for any openings or irritations to the skin. Drying between the toes is especially important to reduce bacteria growth. Bacteria grow well in areas that are dark, warm and moist. Daily foot care also helps increase the flow of healthy blood to the feet, which often need help since they are the furthest point in circulation.

Heel protectors are cupped pads with a firm outside covering to shape them. They are secured to the patient's foot with Velcro straps and can be worn in bed or out. The positioning of the protector on the foot should be checked because they can shift when the patient changes position. A soft pillow or rolled towel can be placed under the patient's ankles when he is lying on his back in bed. This raises the heel off of the bed and reduces pressure and shearing.

Toenails and fingernails should be kept clean and trimmed. A podiatrist who makes house calls may be contacted to perform nail care, especially in patients with diagnosed circulatory problems or who have diseased nails. Care should be taken by the person cutting the nails not to trim too low because the underlying skin can be accidentally cut. This can increase the potential for infection, especially in patients with altered wound healing. In addition, some medications such as steroids can reduce the body's ability to heal or fight infection. The doctor, nurse or pharmacist can make the patient aware of this side effect. Nails should be trimmed when they are warm, such as after bathing, to make cutting easier.

Special nail cutters are available from the pharmacy. Care should be taken to keep finger nails short and clean since patients may scratch themselves with long or uneven nails. Socks can be put on both hands and feet to keep the patient from scratching himself. In addition, bacteria may accumulate under the nails and create an infection, especially if the patient has a rash or scabs that they scratch.

THE FACE

Nose

Care of the patient's nose generally consists of removing any discharge, and keeping the skin intact by keeping it clean and keeping the nails trimmed to avoid scratches.

Remove encrusted drainage with saline nose drops or warm water soaks. Nose drops can be recommended by the doctor and instilled according to bottle directions. A warm, moist compress may also loosen crusting but care should be taken that it is moist, not dripping wet.

During the winter, heated indoor air can draw fluids from the room and from the patient, causing dryness to the mucous membranes of the eyes, nose and mouth. If the home has steam radiators, a pan of water should be kept on top while the radiator while it is being used, and refilled often. This will increase the moisture in the environment as the water in the pan evaporates.

Eyes

Eyes can be washed with a warm, moist washcloth to keep them clean and remove drainage. Eyes should be cleaned from the inner corner to the outer corner to prevent contamination of the tear ducts and eye surfaces. There are also drops available to provide moisture to the eye.

Ears

If the patient has wax buildup in his ears, hearing may be reduced and any medications instilled in the ears may not be absorbed properly. Over-the-counter wax removal systems are available and the doctor can recommend one for use. *Never* insert a cotton swab into the ear canal as damage may result, and wax or other drainage may be packed further into the canal.

SKIN CARE AFTER SURGERY

Sutures or staples in a surgical area or at an injury site can be removed by the nurse at home with a doctor's order. This may allow the patient avoid a trip to the doctor. In rare cases, the nurse may not be able to access all of the staples or sutures.

Then the patient's doctor may need to make a home visit or see the patient in the office so that a local anesthetic can be injected under the skin and the doctor can then probe the site to increase visibility of sutures or staples.

7

INCONTINENCE

Urinary and bowel incontinence requires frequent and effective intervention. The body fluids excreted during these episodes of involuntary release can be irritating to the skin if not removed quickly and properly. Further, incontinence can occur in patients who are aware of what is happening, so discretion and emotional support are critical.

There are many causes of incontinence, including medications, surgery, loss of reflexes, reduction in neurological function or weakening of sphincter muscles due to the aging process. Patients may also suffer from urgency—having the sensation to void or defecate without the ability to get to the bathroom or commode in time. The problem of incontinence may be temporary or permanent, and general care remains the same.

A visiting nurse may institute a regime for incontinence care and reassess it for effectiveness. The patient's special needs, concerns and ability to participate will be considered.

Toileting schedules can be initiated to assist with a patient's needs. For patients who are aware that they are going to pass urine or feces, every effort should be made to get them to a toilet. If a patient develops a routine for bathroom needs, the times that they usually have to go should be communicated to the caregivers. If a patient cannot indicate need but will use the commode if put on it, the patient should be placed on the commode every two hours or according to his own pattern.

Both groups of patients benefit from time spent initially to establish a routine. It has a positive effect on the patient's psychological status, and reduces the potential for skin breakdown.

For patients who have no awareness of passing urine or feces, use of a toileting schedule is not possible. An attempt to remove soiled diapers or underpads and clean the skin should be immediate. Skin should be cleaned with warm soapy water and the caregiver should wear gloves.

WIPES

Disposable wipes can also be used for cleaning up incontinence matter. Although more costly than soap and water, the wipes are easy, moist and some have added skin moisturizing treatments. The wipes are also beneficial for patients using the bathroom or commode, or who use a bed pan. The wipes can increase the surface area cleaned by the patient or caregiver, and provide the patient with a feeling of cleanliness.

PROTECTIVE PRODUCTS

Products that may be used to protect both the patient and bedding from body secretions include underpads, diapers or briefs, and waterproof pads.

A large plastic sheet, shower curtain or tablecloth can be used to cover bedding, but it should not be placed directly next to the patient's skin. Though these plastic coverings provide a barrier to protect the bedding, the moisture that they repel irritates the patients skin and may aid in skin breakdown. Additionally the plastic coverings may increase the patient's sweat production, which also adds moisture and irritation. Plastic barriers are best used when skin can be cleaned and dried immediately.

Heavy cloth squares can be placed under the patient to absorb moisture and drainage while keeping the skin relatively dry. These must be changed and cleaned frequently, however. A heavy terry towel can also provide the necessary absorbency without irritating the skin.

Disposable underpads that have an absorbent side and a plastic side are available. Some insurance companies do not provide coverage for commercial items though because their use can be frequent and costly.

Adult diapers or briefs can absorb moisture and protect the skin. The briefs come in sizes from small to extra large; the package will indicate the weight allowance or hip size that it will accommodate. For patients who have some loss of bladder/bowel control but are still active, products such as children's disposable training pants may be used. However, these have smaller proportions.

Since these types of products are used often, and some insurance plans do not pay for them, expense can be an issue. Many stores sell their own brand of incontinence protection which may be a cost-efficient option, considering that they are disposable. The amount and frequency of incontinence should be assessed when choosing a product because some afford protection for short periods of time but are smaller and more comfortable for the patient.

Changing Diapers

When applying an adult diaper to a bed-bound patient, roll half of the diaper tightly. Place the patient on his or her side and lay the rolled side as far under the patient's backside as possible, leaving the unrolled half flat on the bed. Turn the patient onto the flat side of the diaper and grasp the rolled side of the diaper that is now visible. Do so slowly and reposition the patient to access more of the diaper if needed. If the diaper is pulled hard, the plastic covering may tear, or the inside absorbent layer may pull apart, reducing its effectiveness. The tabs for the diapers go in the back. If applying any ointments or creams prior to the diaper, be sure that fingers are dry when touching the tabs as any residue left on the fingers can coat the tabs and the adhesive may not work. A small towel can be left near the patient during care to wipe fingers.

Soiled diapers and underpads along with the material used for cleaning up should be double-bagged for disposal. In addition to providing infection control, double-bagging reduces odors.

ODOR CONTROL

In addition to double-bagging diapers, pads and waste, there are other methods for removing odors from the patient's area. Deodorizing sprays and preparations, such as diaper pail tablets, can be placed in the garbage can. Lemon scented sprays or deodorizing liquids can be placed in containers around the room, but only use this method if the patient cannot access the liquids and won't mistake them for drinkable solutions. Carpet freshening powder may also help with odor reduction, but be sure to use an odor neutralizer as perfumed powders may only mask odor and may have an overwhelming aroma. Baking soda can be sprinkled into the garbage pail to reduce odor. Deodorized garbage bags are also available.

CREATIVE SOLUTIONS

Creative solutions to incontinence wear are possible and may include the insertion of an adhesive-backed feminine protection pad inside of underwear. Products that are easily removed and disposed of are important for patients who apply and remove their own appliances. Keep an assortment of products available in the home to help meet the patient's needs during random episodes of diarrhea or increased urinary output.

Unique ideas for protecting bedding are always possible. Insert a disposable underpad inside a pillowcase and then use the pillowcase as a pull sheet under a narrow patient. If the patient is more broad, the underpad can be placed between the folds of a flat sheet that is used as a pull sheet.

If the basic principles of skin care are observed—which include keeping the skin clean and dry, and reducing pressure and shearing on the skin—feel free to try whatever solution is appropriate.

CATHETERS

Medications to reduce the flow of urine are available. However, they may stop the flow altogether causing the patient to need a temporary or permanent urinary drainage device such as a Foley catheter. Or if urine contact with the skin is preventing healing or causing skin breakdown, a Foley catheter may be inserted to keep urine away from the skin. Catheters can be inserted and cared for at home with caregiver instruction on how to identify drainage problems, signs of urinary infection and how to keep the catheter clean and infection free.

External catheters that are not invasive are also available to help remove urine and keep the skin clean. For men, the device is applied to the penis much like a condom. It is then attached to a urinary drainage bag. For women, an adhesive-edged plastic bag secures to the outside of the labia and has a drainage tube at the end that diverts urine into a drainage bag. External catheters are more difficult for women to use because a woman's urine is not directed out of the body along a straight path. The urine can stay on fragile perineal skin or can loosen the adhesive, causing the appliance to fall off.

Devices for chronic or very frequent loose stools include rectal tubes that are inserted into the rectum for drainage. This tube only works if the consistency of the stool is thin enough to pass through the tube.

The doctor should be notified of any changes in the color, odor, frequency or amount of urinary or fecal drainage. Further, if there is bleeding, hesitancy or pain with bowel or bladder output, the doctor needs to be notified.

Reducing fluids after dinner can reduce the amount of urine passed at night. For patients who have incontinence during the night, this fluid reduction may reduce or eliminate the problem. Some foods have natural diuretic qualities, such as asparagus and some herbal teas. Avoiding or decreasing the use of these products can also help control urinary output.

Diuretics should be taken early in the morning unless a time is specified by the doctor. If a patient is using diuretics and drastically reduces his amount of fluid intake, the doctor needs to be aware so that measures can be taken to prevent dehydration.

Patients who are independent in the bathroom can use a squeeze bottle filled with warm soapy water to clean hard-to-reach areas in the perineum. The squeeze bottle is helpful for patients with limited manual dexterity because it directs the stream of water. Pre-moistened wipes can also be an effective and easy method for cleaning the perineal area. Avoid the use of perfumed preparations, especially if any openings in the skin are noted. And finally, patients and caregivers should always remember to wash their hands afterwards.

8

CLOTHING

LAYERING

Clothing should be layered with as much use of cotton clothing as possible. Cotton allows for air circulation through the layers and can help keep the patient cool and dry. Likewise, the layers allow warmth to stay between them, keeping the patient warm and can be removed as needed.

Begin with a cotton undershirt, which can be worn instead of a traditional undergarment. Packages of undershirts are sold in department stores. Because styles and availability may vary, it is wise to buy several of a favored garment in order to have them on-hand. Further layers may consist of a long- or short-sleeve T-shirt, button shirt, and a sweater, sweatshirt or vest.

FASTENING

A patient's ability to button, snap and zipper must be assessed when choosing clothing. Garments that open in the front as opposed to those that must be pulled over the head are best. A patient may lose his footing when pulling a garment over his head, or he may have to remember to remove glasses, or he may have to struggle to take the garment off.

Patients who are dependent may benefit from clothes that fasten with Velcro in the back. This allows easier access to the patient's skin on the back and buttocks, as well as easier removal of undergarments. If a dependent patient wears clothing that fastens in front, the back of the garment will be underneath them. This means that the patient will need to be shifted in order to access their backside and the clothing may become tangled or wrinkled, causing the bunched up fabric to increase pressure on the skin.

Catalogues and specialty shops sell clothing designed for bed-bound patients and those who are dependent in self care. However, the patient's garments can be assessed for feasibility of wearing backwards and when possible, adapted by a tailor with the addition of Velcro.

Slacks and undergarments should be easy to open and to lower, especially if urinary frequency or urgency is a problem. Slacks may not be a good choice for some patients because of the difficulty in pulling them up and down. Many department stores carry housecoats that can be used as an alternative garment for women.

SHOES

Shoes with rubber soles that are properly fitted provide the best footwear. The rubber soles should have some traction to reduce slipping. The caregiver should get rid of all shoes that are unsafe or that fit improperly, and may need to do so without the patient's knowledge. Visiting therapists may be able to suggest a specific brand or type of footwear.

If a patient has swelling of the feet, moccasin-type shoes can be used. This footwear accommodates any increase in foot size that may occur during the day, while still maintaining some fashion. Shoes should be tried on at night if swelling is a problem because the foot will be most swollen at the day's end.

If a patient has an alteration in her gait when walking, she may benefit from shoes that tie instead of slip on. Tied shoes or those with Velcro closures help to keep the foot secured in the shoe. Laces made from elastic can make tying easier. Shoe horns, especially with long handles, are helpful for applying footwear.

Lightweight shoes may be needed for patients with reduced strength because the added weight of a heavy shoe can lead to difficulty lifting the foot.

UNDERGARMENTS

Underwear bottoms or pantyhose that come in contact with the patient's perineal area should be made from cotton. This allows moisture to be wicked away from the skin in an area where bacteria can easily grow.

Restrictive leg apparel (socks, pantyhose, leggings, etc.) should be avoided because of their potential to reduce circulation. White cotton socks are the best choice for their ability to absorb moisture and because white socks do not contain dyes that can irritate the skin.

Socks should be applied to the feet and then gently pulled up at the toes to reduce the pressure on the tips of the toes. If a patient has long or sharp toe nails, the pressure can bend the nail causing pressure at the base of the nail, or it can cause irregular edges to dig into the soft tissue of the toes.

OTHER TIPS

- Hems on any apparel should be kept above the patient's shoes to avoid tripping.
- Belts may restrict comfortable motion if worn too tightly. Suspenders are a reasonable alternative if clothing needs to be supported on the patient's frame.
- Be sure to check return policies when buying special items: though stores that provide patient care products may be more understanding of a caregiver who is purchasing for a patient who may not appreciate their choices, they are likewise more aware of potential contact with body fluids while the items are being tried on.
- Special order items are almost never returnable once they leave the store.
- Reduced activity and medications such as blood thinners (prescribed or OTC such as aspirin) can change temperature perception and acclimation. Dress the patient in layers more according to their comfort than to outdoor temperatures. However, t'he caregiver's judgement and insistence may be needed during extreme temperatures or when the patient must go outdoors.
- Used clothing in good condition may be donated to local nursing homes, especially items that are easy to take on and off.

9

COMMUNICATION

INTERNAL COMMUNICATIONS

It is extremely important to have communication between all caregivers, family members and advocates in the home. Patient routines, preferences, appointments, medications, and status changes need to be relayed to all members of the home care team. This chapter will discuss ways to establish and maintain good communication.

Using a Calendar

Obtain a large calendar that can be used as the communication center. Locate it in an area that is frequently used and where it is easily readable. The kitchen refrigerator is a good location, or on a message-type board. The calendar should have large squares so that all the information can be legibly recorded. Charts can be broken down into three sections: day (7 a.m. to 3 p.m.); evening (3 p.m. to 11 p.m.); and night (11 p.m. to 7 a.m.).

Scheduling

Information that should be placed on the calendar includes: appointments with doctors, nurses, therapists or other ancillary services; scheduled visits of family and friends; and medications that are stopped and/or restarted on specific dates. Lab work schedules can also be indicated, especially if the patient has to avoid food and drink prior to testing.

Marking the date and time of scheduled nursing or therapist visits helps avoid over-scheduling for patients that tire easily. Appointments can be arranged for days or times that are compatible with the patient's energy levels. Keep in mind, however, that a nurse or therapist submits a plan that includes the frequency of visits needed for each week and they are expected to follow this schedule. Missed visits are documented on the patient's record with explanation. The insurance company may refuse to continue coverage if visits are frequently missed or refused for social obligations. Visits should not be re-scheduled due to lunch dates or hair appointments.

Vital Signs

Patient information that can be documented on the calendar includes: blood sugar results for diabetic patients; blood pressure readings if done by the caregiver or nurse; temperature; and bowel movements or amounts of urinary output. In the same area, separate sheets with turning schedules and fluid or food intake can be posted. If this type of information is recorded in one location, it can be brought with the patient to a doctor visit or checked by the visiting nurse. Caregivers can use these records to determine patient care during their time on duty.

Recording bowel movements may help identify patterns of elimination that would be treated unnecessarily if not documented as routine. For example, a patient that consistently eliminates every three or four days may not need intervention for constipation, while a patient who has a bowel movement at irregular intervals may need changes in diet or addition of medication or fluids. If the nurse visits twice a week, the caregiver may not be able to recall the last bowel movement, or it may have occurred when a different caregiver was present. If that information is not communicated, the nurse may contact the doctor for intervention that might be unnecessary. Similarly, by documenting the fluids or food a patient has taken, dietary requirements or restrictions can be met.

Emergency Information

Some of the most important information that should be listed on the calendar includes: the names and numbers of those responsible for making decisions for the patient, especially those who are named in advance directives; doctors and ancillary care givers; the patient's current medication regime; and any allergies that the patient may have. This information may be critical if a medical emergency arises. It will enable the ambulance crew and emergency room staff to have complete information that can hasten medical treatment. If a patient has a directive for resuscitation, it should be posted as well. This can prevent the implementation of emergency care if the patient has opted against it.

PATIENT COMMUNICATION

For those patients with visual impairments, written communication should be done using a heavy marker and large print. Large-faced clocks, usually digital, are useful for patients with poor eyesight. Some clocks have the added feature of a push-button that will announce the time.

Erasable boards, chalk boards or children's plastic drawing toys are a method for communicating with patients who cannot talk due to medical condition or fatigue. They are also a technique to plan the day with the patient. Leave it where the patient can refer to it throughout the day.

TELECOMMUNICATION

Telephones can be programmed with frequently used numbers and emergency agencies. Information provided with the phone will help with the programming process. For patients who have trouble remembering which button dials which number, pictures can be taped to the buttons to assist the patient's recall. Large-button phones are easier for patients with decreased manual dexterity or vision.

Telephone bells that will ring in the bathroom or other rooms which do not have a phone can be installed by an electrician. This will alert the patient to phone calls. Portable phones can be used, but reception may be poor and the phone must be placed correctly in the base for recharging. Finally, the volume of the phone receiver and ringer can be amplified for those patients who have trouble hearing.

MASS MEDIA

Sources of media for impaired patients include large print puzzles and books, audiobooks on tape, or headsets that can attach to the television or radio and be worn by the patient. This is especially useful if the patient is hard of hearing, because the volume can be turned up as high as necessary for the patient, without disturbing others in the home or neighbors.

Patients may enjoy having books or magazines read to them, or dictating letters to friends or family. Some volunteer agencies may provide people who enjoy performing these tasks. Libraries often offer books on tape for borrowing.

10

MOBILITY

Alterations in the patient's ability to walk or transfer from one position to another are some of the most common reasons for home care services. A change in the patient's activity tolerance leads to an increase in dependence on others for care.

The nurse will assess each patient's activity and endurance, regardless of the diagnosis on referral. A referral for physical or occupational therapy can be made for new medical conditions, for old ones that limit the patient's activity, or for gradual changes that result in a reduced ability to walk or transfer.

AROUND THE HOUSE

Patients who have had any type of orthopedic surgery may need the services of a visiting nurse for medical intervention, and a therapist to instruct in exercises to help increase activity and flexibility. Patients may be discharged from the hospital with adaptive devices for ambulation that they are using incorrectly or not at all. The therapist will assess the patient's current use of any such devices and then instruct them in their proper use.

If a patient is not currently using a device, he may have one ordered for him and then instructed in its use. The therapist may also discuss with the doctor the possibility of changing to a different device that would be better used by the patient at home. The therapist will also instruct how to use the device in more complex tasks such as climbing stairs and walking on uneven surfaces, which are sometimes encountered outside.

Patients may need more than one device, each to be used in different circumstances such as when the patient is feeling tired or weak, or when the patient is on uneven ground. Occasionally, two of the same device are recommended, such as a walker for use on the upper level of a patient's home, and another for the ground floor. This reduces the need for the patient to carry the walker upstairs or downstairs with them.

Insurance coverage and potential payment for equipment will be discussed with the patient before it is ordered by the nurse or therapist. The patient should fully understand the cost of the item, the expected insurance coverage and the amount that the patient will be expected to pay. If it is an item that many insurance companies refuse to cover, or decide coverage only after examining medical records, the patient should be aware of this before agreeing to have it delivered.

Nursing interventions for patients with altered activity levels include an assessment of how the changes affect the patient's ability to care for himself. If assistance is needed with personal care or medication administration, a referral for help or implementation of a home care plan will be made.

The nurse will determine whether the patient is performing any exercises that the therapist has provided, and the patient's ability to do so. Patients should be encouraged to pace their activities and to take frequent, scheduled breaks. For patients who are unsteady on their feet, the caregiver will be taught how to supervise or assist the patient when walking.

An apron can be tied to the front of a walker to give the patient a place to store personal items while walking, and to keep the patient's hands free to hold the walker. If used, the apron strings should be kept short to prevent tripping. Commercial products designed especially for walkers are available, but they may be costly.

In the event of a patient fall at home that does not result in injury but leaves the patient unable to return to bed unassisted, the local police may be notified and attend to help the patient back to bed. If a patient sustains a fall and has any pain, unnatural body position, or loss of consciousness with or prior to the fall, an ambulance should be called to make an assessment and transfer the patient to the hospital as needed.

Hairdressers who make home visits are available, or the patient's usual beautician may offer to come to the patient's home. Care should be taken to avoid sustained chemical contact for the patient because breathing the fumes from some hair care products can make the patient feel ill or increase respiratory effort. The patient's ability to maintain a position with their head extended into a sink for hair washing should be assessed and avoided if not easily tolerated.

Seat lift chairs are available for installation in a patient's home. These allow the patient to change floors as needed. Seat lift chairs run along tracks that are installed directly into the wall along the stairs. The patient sits on the seat at the top or bottom of the stairs, engages the motor and the chair slowly moves the patient along the track. Seatbelts are provided and recommended to reduce falls. These chairs need to be installed by the manufacturer and can be costly. In some homes, installation is not possible because of the stair's design. However, if the arrangements can be made, they are a valuable transportation device within the home.

Establishing a routine should incorporate rest periods which can be sitting with the feet elevated as opposed to going to bed or sleeping. The patients energy levels should be assessed when making routines to incorporate increased activity at times when the patients energy levels are the highest.

OUTSIDE THE HOME

Patients may need to make routine doctor visits, especially if the doctor does not make house calls. For patients who enjoy these trips, every effort should be made to extend the length of the outing if they can tolerate it. A trip to a store or a stop for lunch can help increase the patient's self esteem.

For some patients, getting out may mean simply sitting on a porch or in a yard. If the doctor allows such activity, leaving the home for periods of time can provide mental stimulation and increased activity that may allow the patient to sleep or eat better.

Direct sunlight is contraindicated for some patients because of medications they are taking. The pharmacist will advise of this restriction. Sunblock or a hat can be worn by patients who have sun-sensitive skin as a result of medication or disease process. The patient can also be shielded with an umbrella or sit in a shady area.

Transportation to scheduled appointments can be arranged by the patient or caregiver. Different types of transportation include automobile, ambulance, taxi, bus, hospital van or senior citizen service with scheduled times and destinations. The patient's ability to get to the curb for pick up, enter the vehicle unassisted or with minimal help, and to keep track of the time for return trips will determine the type of transportation.

If the patient uses a wheelchair, determine if he has to bring his own or if one will be provided by the transportation service. If the patient is not allowed to bring a wheelchair, make certain that there is one available at the destination.

Likewise, if the caregiver is not allowed to travel with the patient, plans to meet at the appointment should be carefully coordinated. Some types of service may allow a caregiver to accompany the patient on outings or may charge a fee for the caregiver. Some communities provide discounted vouchers for senior citizens to use for taxi service, but may limit the quantity allowed. Arrangements for transportation should be made as soon as the doctor appointment is made because seating may be limited.

If a patient is receiving scheduled treatments on an outpatient basis, such as radiation or wound care, the doctor's office or health care facility may arrange transportation. It is in the facility's best interest to provide transportation because it has the patient's care scheduled into a time slot. This continuity of care enables the facility to provide care to many patients without having to factor in those patients who are late or who miss visits due to transportation.

Local senior citizen groups, hospital discharge planners or social workers can provide information about patient transportation services. Some hospitals have buses or vans available as a community service to bring the patients to the hospital for planned lab work, therapy or other treatments. Use of such a facility may become the best choice, even if it is not the patient's primary hospital.

Handicapped license plates or placards are available through the state's department of motor vehicles with provision of proper documentation. Generally, a form must be filled out by the doctor indicating that the patient has medical limitations.

Vacation travel is possible if planning is thorough. Airports, bus terminals and railroads provide access, special boarding accommodations and advocates for patients who are in wheelchairs, or have other medical needs. Plan on arriving at the dispatch site early and asking for help to meet the patient's needs.

Arrangements for patients who are traveling alone must include consideration of the destination and for the return trip. The patient's ticket should be kept with him. Transportation staff should be made aware that the patient is on the trip. This reduces a patient's frustration, especially in crowded areas.

Always take medication in carry-on luggage that will be kept with the patient or companion throughout the entire trip. A copy of all prescriptions should be with the patient, in case a refill is needed, unless the patient's pharmacy has national branches that can access this information.

Pre-filled syringes of injectable medication such as insulin can travel with the patient if the proper containers and refrigeration are provided. Always store the syringes with the plunger facing up to reduce accidental discharge of the medication during travel. Hard plastic toothbrush holders are the best way to store syringes for travel. Ice packs can be used to keep medicine at a cool temperature. Thermal insulated bags will help retain moisture accumulation and coolness.

Supplies needed for wound care should be accessible and also transported in the patient's carry-on luggage along with medication. This is important in case of lost or misplaced luggage.

EXTENDED VISITS

Patients can be referred for home care service, either to provide care or to monitor medical conditions, at the site they are visiting. The agency making the referral will need to know where the patient will be staying, who will be responsible for the patient and for providing care, and who will be the doctor to care for the patient at the destination. If the patient is making a weekend trip, they probably will not need a referral to a new doctor.

Extended visits or ones without scheduled return dates will indicate the need for the patient to have a doctor available to assess and treat if needed. Often, the doctor of the family member that the patient is visiting may agree to be the responsible doctor.

If there is not a doctor available, the patient or family can call the local hospital and obtain a referral. The doctor may request medical records be sent with the patient especially if care is complex or the visit will be lengthy.

Arrangements for medical equipment can be made by the agency to which the patient is referred. It is recommended that items such as wheelchairs, crutches or other ambulatory devices be borrowed if possible. Insurance companies that pay for medical equipment rental may be unable to provide payment for supplies in other sites, especially if the insurance company contracts with suppliers. These details should be considered and plans made before the patient finalizes any other plans for the trip.

CAR TRIPS

If traveling by car, the patient should sit in the back seat with her feet elevated on the seat unless medically contraindicated. Seat belts are especially important because the patient's ability to adapt her body to sudden changes in momentum may be limited by age or medical status

Extended trips that require a patient to be in a position with her legs down can contribute to discomfort, cramps, and swelling in the legs and feet. Road trips should include scheduled stops for bathroom needs, meals and medication administration, as well as the chance to stretch muscles and re-position as needed.

11

THE FORGETFUL PATIENT

Special consideration should be given when deciding whether to care for a forgetful patient at home. A common home care situation arises when a patient is independent enough to walk around, get dressed and verbalize likes and dislikes, but is consistently or irregularly forgetful. The family or advocate agonizes over taking the patient's freedom and independence away by institutionalizing him, but is concerned for the patient's safety if he is allowed to stay at home.

Planning for this patient will depend on caregiver involvement to the extent that the patient needs and will allow help. If a patient becomes dangerous to himself or others, placement may be the only choice. Candid discussion of the patient's mental status should take place with the doctor, along with caregiver's concerns for the feasibility of safe and effective care at home. Clergy, doctor, social worker, family and friends can give support and assist in the decision making.

If placement is the plan, the patient's status regarding independence in activities, understanding of placement, medical condition and insurance coverage will be assessed. The doctor will be able to provide the medical documentation, and a nurse that has received the proper training for the placement assessment will obtain the rest of the information. Contact a visiting nurse agency for information regarding the paperwork necessary for the placement process. The fee to have the placement paperwork done is not often covered by insurance when done at home, but may be covered if done from the hospital.

If a patient is scheduled to be discharged from the hospital, and the family or caregivers feel they cannot provide adequate home care for the patient after being advised of the patient's needs, a discharge planner or social worker will be able to discuss the alternatives such as long- or short-term placement. If the forgetful patient is to be cared for at home, the following information should be helpful.

FORGETFUL VS. CONFUSED

In this text, forgetful and confused patients are grouped for the sake of nursing interventions. On a daily basis, the forgetful patient may not be able to recall his address or dog's name, while the confused patient may believe that it is 1965 or that the person caring for her is a long-since deceased sister. Both changes in mental status may occur for short or extended periods of time, or be related to specific triggers such a time, place or person. Mental changes may also be a side effect of medication, an indicator of dehydration or other change in body chemistry, part of a diagnosed disease process, or the result of the aging process where blood vessels that supply the oxygen-rich blood to the brain have narrowed.

THE NEED FOR IDENTIFICATION

Labels in the patient's clothing that include name, address and phone number can help a patient retrieve his belongings if he is in a day care facility. They can also be used to identify the patient if he wanders away from the home and is unable to find his way back. For this reason, labels should be clearly written and easily located. The same information should be kept on a card in the patient's wallet, purse or pocket. If a patient regularly visits a grocery store, religious facility or hairdresser, this information should be communicated to the proprietor.

If taking a forgetful patient to an organized event in an arena or hall, the seat ticket should be placed in the patient's pocket so that he can be returned to his seat if he wanders away or becomes confused. Identification bracelets can be obtained that contain the patient's diagnosis and allergies, in case of an accident or medical crisis requiring intervention.

COMMUNITY SERVICES

Local police departments should have a recent picture of the confused or forgetful patient. In the event that the patient wanders off, he or she will be easier to recognize. Some police departments offer fingerprint and photo ID cards that are kept on file in local area for identification of lost children. Many will provide the same service for adults with a potential for, or history of, wandering.

Police and fire departments should be aware if a patient is forgetful, especially if there are times that the patient is left alone. If an emergency arises, the rescue process will be faster if the police or fire department knows to look for a patient who may be hiding because they are confused. If the agency is aware that the patient should be in the home, they will know to look for the patient who might not otherwise call for help or respond to the emergency teams verbal search.

Local emergency rooms should also have patient information for recognition if the patient is brought in. At times, the police will bring a confused and wandering patient to the local emergency room for evaluation if there is no way to identify him. They will try to assess if the patient has a medical cause for the confusion, and hopefully someone will recognize the person as a patient. Further, if a family member or caregiver finds that a patient is missing, they may call the hospital to check if the patient was injured. These interventions apply for the area in which a patient resides, as well as any homes where the patient may stay for extended periods of time, such as when care is rotated among children in different geographical locations.

RESISTING CARE

Sometimes, forgetful and confused patients will resist caregivers. In this case, every effort should be made to install the caregiver in the home in a non-threatening manner.

Creative ways to use caregivers when patients are opposed to help might be to tell the patient that the person is there to perform housework. If the patient becomes familiar with the caregiver, he may then allow the person to assist him with personal needs. Paid caregivers of the same gender as the patient are usually the most acceptable to the patient and therefore, the most effective.

All approaches to a forgetful or confused patient should be slow and gentle. Any person who approaches the patient quickly or forcefully may frighten the patient and increase his resistance to care or supervision.

A patient who resists any aspect of personal care should not be forced to accept it at that time. Offering to help with care may be more agreeable to the patient at a later time, even without specific changes in the approach.

If a patient refuses care that would be detrimental to his health or welfare if omitted, the family or caregiver must seek intervention. Examples include patients who refuse all medications, food, bathing or assistance when walking despite the fact that they are unsafe when doing it alone. The doctor may need to prescribe medications to relax the patient to reduce his resistance. This does not mean that the patient will become docile or lose his independence because of the medication. Some types of medication can simply make the patient less suspicious or combative, and allow an easier approach by caregivers.

Reasoning with a confused or forgetful patient may be frustrating for the caregiver, who feels that she is making the need for care clear to the patient. It is even more frustrating when the caregiver is a grown child or other family member who remembers the patient's previous intelligence and dignity. This situation may require the intervention of a counselor or health professional who can best teach about the disease process and how it affects the patient's reasoning ability.

REASONING WITH THE PATIENT

Some diseases such as brain tumors or strokes can render a patient emotionally labile, angry, aggressive or apathetic—which may be a drastic personality change. An explanation by the doctor or nurse regarding the areas of the brain that were affected, and the behavior changes that can be anticipated, allows the caregiver to prepare emotionally for the patient's response.

Patients can lose the ability to recognize or remember people who are close to them, or special dates and events from the past. Family members may feel that if they just try hard enough and in the right manner, they will restore the patient's memory. These attempts can prove comforting to some family caregivers, especially when they see what they interpret as recall or recognition. At other times the attempts increase the caregivers' frustration. Caregivers sometimes focus on these attempts to reduce their own feelings of inadequacy regarding participation in patient care. Attempts at re-orientation should never be discouraged if the caregiver feels that she is helping. Patients should be assessed to determine if they are becoming more confused by orientation attempts, which can be limited to shorter periods of time.

For caregivers who feel helpless regarding a patient's inability to recall time, place or person, they may feel helpful if they make flashcards for the patient, with the date or the patient's address. Toy stores also offer an assortment of bright pictures and words on cards that may be used to stimulate the patient's intellect. Though these may seem like juvenile exercises, patients may respond positively to objects that they can recognize.

It is a common tendency to ask a patient to recall a detail from his past with the hopes that, if the patient is told a fact about himself, he will then integrate it into his life. An example would be to say to the patient, "You always loved crossword puzzles, don't you remember?" However, this might not work and the person who offered the information will be frustrated if she does not see a spark of recognition by the patient. A more appropriate approach may be to give the patient a puzzle and help him do it. If the patient shows interest, the caregiver can then remind him that he liked this activity.

SUPERVISION

Small alterations to the patient's environment can improve the caregiver's supervision of the patient's activities, without reducing privacy or independence. However, for forgetful and confused patients, the environment should not be drastically rearranged. Any changes that are made should be clearly explained to the patient as often as needed to provide reassurance and allow participation.

Doors can be cut in half so that the top half is left open for visualization of the patient. This is also a way to keep the patient confined to his room if he is unsafe leaving the room unassisted.

If a patient refuses a half door, or if it is too extreme or costly, a peephole can be installed in the door with the lens reversed. This allows the caregiver to look into the room and observe the patient without the patient being aware or disturbed. Another option, as mentioned in a previous chapter, is a baby monitor. This will allow the caregiver to hear what is going on in the room, and be alerted to the sounds of objects falling or cries for help.

Bells can be placed on doors so that, when a patient leaves the room or home, the ringing bell can alert the caregiver to the patient's location and intention. Battery-operated doorbells or a bike horn can be placed near the patient so that they have an easy method to contact the caregiver if needed.

Gates can be used at patient doors or staircases to deter the patient. Some patients will try to climb over them, which can result in injury, so they must be used at the caregiver's discretion.

A key to the front door should be left with a neighbor or advocate who is easily accessible and nearby. The police should be aware of who holds this key in the event of an emergency. If the patient lives in a multi-unit building, the superintendent should be able to provide entry into the patient's home.

Leaving Notes

Notes can be placed on doors to remind the patient not to leave. Similarly, a note may be placed in the kitchen to remind the patient to turn off the gas or water, or in other rooms to remind the patient to turn off lights or lock doors. If a patient needs frequent reminders, this may indicate that the patient needs more supervision.

In The Kitchen

As an additional safety precaution in the kitchen, take the knobs off the stove and oven controls. This will prevent the patient from turning on the oven or stove if she forgets that it is a prohibited activity.

Nighttime

Nighttime can be especially difficult when caring for the confused or forgetful patient. If a patient requires supervision during the night, a second caregiver (formal or informal) must be considered to provide relief. Every attempt should be made to prevent patients from sleeping excessively during the day so that they will be able to sleep at night. Using planned activities or rousing the patient from frequent naps during the day can help establish better sleeping habits. Additionally, evening routines such as playing a radio instead of television can help facilitate sleep. As with children, eliminating shows that are violent or action-oriented two hours before bed can help produce more restful sleeping.

Nighttime wandering can be extremely unsafe, especially if the patient goes into the kitchen. If a patient routinely wakes and goes into the kitchen for a snack or drink, leave one out on the table for him. Baby monitors are especially helpful at night to alert the caregiver of a wandering patient. Check packages for recommended distance between monitor and receiver, especially if using them on different floors of the house.

MEDICATIONS

All medications that are not being used should be removed from the patient's access. Alarm clocks can be set to remind the patient that he needs to take his medication. Phone calls from family or friends can be used for the same purpose

With forgetful and confused patients, medication administration should be closely supervised. In the event of suspected misuse of medication, the doctor should be notified. If the patient shows signs of altered physical status such as lethargy, increased confusion, nausea, vomiting or labored breathing and chest pains, emergency intervention is indicated. In some cases, pills may be counted to determine whether the patient is taking his medication as directed. If a pill count indicates misuse, intervention is needed. If the patient shows any signs of overdose or medication reaction, the doctor will need to know which medication is suspected of causing the symptoms—again, a pill count based on the date of prescription pickup may help. The vial should indicate the date the prescription was filled and the quantity of pills included. If the fill date was 3 days ago for 30 once-daily pills, and the vial only has 10 pills remaining, the conclusion can be that this pill was overused.

DRIVING

Car keys should be placed away from patient access if the patient is unable to drive because of physical or mental disability. Forgetful patients may not recall being told not to drive, or they may think that it is okay to drive a short distance. If the patient is able to understand, clearly explain that driving is no longer possible and offer to take the patient where he would have previously taken himself, or arrange alternate transportation.

For patients who can no longer drive, suggesting outings with them may reduce their feeling of dependence while allowing them a feeling of freedom at getting out of the house. Ask the patient to accompany you while you run your errands, then when already out, suggest that the patient may want to stop somewhere for herself. This enables the patient to feel less burdensome if they are doing you the favor of keeping you company.

If a patient is irrational regarding the loss of driving privileges, explain that driving is restricted because of the doctor's orders. This may transfer the patient's anger to the doctor and allow the caregiver to continue a good relationship with the patient.

Driving restrictions are important for the confused patient because not only may they forget where they where going and how to get there, but they may have decreased response times to other drivers' actions which increases the potential for accident and injury. This may occur especially at night when visibility is limited

95

and light from other cars distracting. Some patients may have restrictions imposed for nighttime driving only which may be agreeable to them.

12

WHEN TO SEEK MEDICAL INTERVENTION

The following is a list of problems that may occur that require medical intervention. However, in general, any symptoms or complaints that are persistent or severe should be told to the doctor. If the doctor is not available, the patient should be taken to the emergency room.

If questions arise about which medications should be taken by the patient, or what to do if doses are missed, hold further medication administration and contact the doctor. Tell the doctor exactly which medications where missed or overused and by how many doses or tablets. Doctors generally would rather be contacted to discuss questions and reduce complications, than have a medical crisis arise.

FINDING A DOCTOR

Doctors are committed to caring for their patients. They should not give the patient or caregiver the impression that they are being disturbed by questions. If this situation arises, the patient may find it necessary to change doctors.

When either seeking a new doctor or going to another doctor for a consultation, the patient can request a copy of his medical record from the original doctor. It may be easier for the patient to bring this record to the new doctor, than for him to try to recall his entire medical history. The records can be obtained by writing to the former doctor and asking her to release the records.

The doctor may send the records to the new or consulting doctor, or may forward them to the patient. If records are extensive, the doctor's office may have a policy that requests a fee from the patient to cover the cost of copying.

If a patient's primary doctor refers the patient to another doctor for a consultation, the doctor making the referral will generally contact the consulting doctor and tell him about the patient's medical history and why the referral is being made. Insurance companies that function under primary care may only approve consultations that originate from the primary doctor, including even routine consults to eye or ear doctors.

BODY SYSTEMS

The following information is presented by body systems and is very general. The doctor should advise the patient and caregiver of any expected side effects of treatment or the disease process, what the doctor wants to be notified about, and when the patient should seek emergency care.

Eyes

Seek care for any changes in vision including flashing lights, dark or floating spots, halo vision, or a loss or reduction of vision. Also seek care for the following conditions: redness, pain or irritation to the eyes; onset of drainage especially if it is bloody, green/yellow or foul smelling; and any blunt or traumatic injury.

Ears

Medical intervention is recommended for any: ringing in the ears; dull or sharp ear pains; loss of hearing; drainage from the ears of any kind; inflammation of the outer or inner ear; and insertion of any objects into the ear that cannot be retrieved from the outer ear.

Nose

Seek medical attention for: nasal drainage caused by colds or allergies that is not relieved with traditional means; green/yellow or foul smelling drainage; crusting of drainage that inhibits breathing; frequent or recurrent expulsion of fluids through the nose that are taken in by mouth; and bleeding from the nose especially by those taking blood thinners.

Mouth

Seek care for: open sores in the mouth or on the lips or gums; thick/dry tongue; bleeding from the mouth or gums; difficulty swallowing that is not relieved with sips of fluid or use of thickeners; choking on foods or fluids that results in the patient turning blue (cyanotic); complaints of sore throat; and tooth decay that may need removal of affected teeth.

Head

Headaches require medical attention if they: are not relieved with conventional or prescribed means; become worse when in direct light or with position change; are accompanied by dizziness or ringing in the ears; occur with neck pain or inability to turn the head; occur with loss of consciousness or confusion; happen after a fall with head injury; are accompanied by persistent or severe nosebleeds; occur with fevers/chills.

Mental Status

A change in the patient's mental status that is sudden or severe, without diagnosed potential for the same, should be brought to the doctor's attention. Other situations that indicate the need for medical intervention would include: irrational or inappropriate behavior; combative or uncontrollable episodes, especially when the caregiver is at risk for injury; any change in the level of consciousness that leaves the patient hard to awaken; increases in restlessness or sleepiness that are not anticipated; and any seizure-like activity involving uncontrolled movement of the body, flailing of arms or legs, alternating periods of rigidity and muscle relaxation.

Neurological

Seek medical intervention for any: changes in the patient's sensation in his hands and feet; numbness or tingling in the body; headaches or dizziness; slurred speech; difficulty expressing words or thoughts; weakness to one side of the body; facial drooping; lack of coordination of facial muscles, especially that results in drooling, or in any other muscle groups; inability to grasp an object and hold it; inability to follow directions to perform a specific movement or task; and any change in mental status regarding orientation to time, place, person, day and date.

Heart and Lungs

Immediate medical intervention is necessary for any episodes of chest pain or palpitations that are new in occurrence or do not respond to prescribed medications. Also seek immediate care for any: shortness of breath or rapid breathing that is not relieved with rest or controlled breathing; shortness of breath that occurs with chest pains/palpitations; coughing or wheezing that does not respond to prescribed medications; coughing that produces green/yellow drainage or blood; and fever and chills with respiratory symptoms.

Gastrointestinal

Seek care for sustained episodes of nausea or vomiting, especially if they occur after medical treatment is in effect, and for vomiting of blood, fecal matter or dark material with the consistency of coffee grounds. Medical intervention is also required if a patient refuses or is unable to eat or take in fluids.

Bowel movements that are severally irregular, either frequent or infrequent, should prompt medical intervention, as well as: bowel movements that are bloody, frothy, contain undigested foods, are painful or have stopped; that are tar-like, black in color and cannot be attributed to iron or other medication use.

Seek care if the patient's abdomen is hard, painful to touch or has increased noticeably in size unrelated to the patient's pattern of bowel movements or meals. Any guarding of abdomen by the patient, or refusal to turn to either side because of pain, should also be reason to seek medical care.

Genitourinary

Medical intervention is indicated for frequent urination that is not related to fluid intake or medication use, or that is accompanied by burning or pain. Other symptoms that require medical care include: difficulty initiating or maintaining the flow of urine; a complete lack of urine output; a foul odor to urine that is unrelated to hydration status; mucous or blood in the urine; swelling, redness or itching of perineal tissues with or without vaginal drainage; the appearance of soft tissue protruding into the vaginal opening or in the urethra; or the passage of stools through the urethra, or of urine via rectum.

Muscular

Consult a doctor if the patient: lacks the ability to change position or move his limbs; has pain or an unnatural position of a limb; has a fall that result in pain, unnatural position or inability to move a limb; has a loss of manual dexterity; has continued pain or soreness to a specific muscle or muscle group; is suddenly unable to move about when he was previously ambulatory without other specific complaints.

Skin

Medical attention is recommended for: new onsets of open areas or sores; burns; skin that is red, tender, swollen, or has red streaking; drainage from an existing wound that becomes green/yellow or foul smelling; the onset of rashes or other skin irritations that are hot, itchy, draining or blistered.

Wounds that are not responding to the prescribed treatments or are getting larger should be brought to a doctor's attention. The doctor should also be consulted about: open skin in areas that are not exposed to pressure such as the breasts or abdomen; poor healing of incision(s); incisions that open up; and sutures or staples at an incision site that become dislodged, painful or irritated.

Seek care for any: bruising that is not attributable to injury especially in patients that are taking blood thinners; changes in the patient's skin color to pale or dusky, or any cyanosis, especially if patient's skin becomes cold and clammy; and frequent or sustained blue hue to lips or nailbeds.

Circulation

Consult a physician for the following symptoms: any loss of sensation including numbness or tingling to hands or feet that is not an expected effect of medication, disease or aging; any body area that suddenly becomes cold, dusky in color, or loses feeling, mobility and function; and any increased swelling of the feet or other body parts that exceeds expected amounts, is new in occurrence, or does not respond to medication.

EMERGENCIES

If a medical emergency arises, the doctor may advise transport to the hospital. The following information describes the aspects of emergency intervention that the patient and caregiver need to know.

Emergency transportation to a hospital can be accessed by calling 911 or the local emergency response number. Some insurance companies will not pay for trips to the emergency room that do not result in a patient admission. Others will determine payment on a case-by-case basis. While ambulance service can be costly, it should not be a determining factor in use, especially in an emergency situation.

It is important for caregivers and family members to know which hospital or medical center the local ambulance will take the patient. Policies regarding transportation destination are made by the ambulance company and generally, the patient is taken to the nearest facility that can meet his needs. In the event that the hospital is not one at which the patient's doctor practices, the patient can be stabilized and, if possible, transferred to the hospital of choice. If a patient requires a service that is available at a specialized facility, such as burn unit or trauma center, the ambulance may be directed to take the patient directly there.

To find out where a patient was taken, it may be easier to contact the police who attend emergency calls or the ambulance service. Calling local emergency rooms can be frustrating and time consuming, and some facilities may prohibit the release of patient information over the phone.

Regarding cellular or car phones, when 911 is dialed, a state operator takes the call. They are not aware of the town that you are calling from, so be as specific as possible when giving information. The operator will need to know what street you are on, the cross road and the town that you are in. If on a highway, they will need to know the nearest exit and the direction that you are traveling. Giving this information quickly and correctly will enhance the response time.

Emergency access devices are available for home care. Part of the electronic system is worn by the patient, and part is attached to the patient's phone system. If the patient needs medical help, she can press the button on the small box that she wears on a necklace. The monitoring company is alerted and calls the patient. If there is no answer, the company will dispatch police or ambulance to the patient. Also on record with a monitoring agency would be a key holder, who would be contacted to allow the emergency personnel to gain access to the patient's home. The obvious problem with this system is that the patient must be able to access the device.

Using regularly scheduled callers to check on the patient also helps alert family and friends to a patient's unexpected needs. Again, the patient must be able to answer the phone.

If there is no plan for regular patient contact or use of emergency alert devices, a neighbor can alert family or police if a patient deviates from routine. Some basic indicators would include excess accumulation of mail or newspapers, or lights being left on. For patients who are forgetful, these signs may inconclusive.

If an emergency service arrives to find a patient alone and in need of medical attention, visible information in the home can hasten treatment. A medication list including allergies may allow for treatment in the home and make a hospital trip unnecessary, such as for diabetic patients. Having a list of doctors and family members to be contacted is also good because the emergency response team can communicate with them and possibly get more information about the patient. Listing recent hospitalizations and reasons may also help the response team.

The use of medical bracelets, cards or necklaces can make the patient's medical diagnoses known and enhance treatment. Information is important, especially if the patient has communication deficits such as hearing or vision loss. The patient can then be approached properly to facilitate treatment. The information may also explain an unusual symptom that would have caused the emergency worker to provide unnecessary treatment.

A copy of the patient's health care directive that is clearly visible can reduce the initiation of life-saving measures. Appropriate comfort measures can be taken if the patient is actively dying.

If the patient has a frequent need for emergency care, have a bag packed with necessary personal items. These types of patients are carefully considered when being referred for home care.

If the caregiver is accessing emergency services, he should make the call from a phone near the patient. This will allow the emergency operator to offer advice, obtain information to help the response team, verify directions to the patient's location and reassure the caregiver that help is nearby. Close proximity to the patient is also important because if the patient's condition improves while the response team is in route, they can slow down the speed with which they are responding and reduce the risk that they take when driving.

If the emergency operator terminates the call after taking all pertinent information, the caregiver should stay calm and comfort the patient if able. This is not always possible because of the caregiver's personal response to emergencies.

The patient may be difficult for the caregiver to look at if bloody or severely ill, or if access to the patient's location is limited or impossible.

The caregiver can wait outside if the home is difficult to find, or a neighbor can do this. Turn on outside lights, especially those that illuminate the house number, to speed response. If the house does not have a number on it, or the numbers don't run in order, alert the operator to this fact when placing the call.

While the emergency team is in route, the caregiver can also use this time to collect the patient's belongings, to call family members or to collect important patient information that the response team may need. The caregiver should also find the patient's insurance card to be able to provide information to the hospital as needed.

The caregiver may need to provide information about the events leading up to the crisis, including patient complaints, unusual foods that were eaten, falls or injuries in the recent past, desires that the patient may have verbalized regarding hurting himself, new medications taken by the patient, or the possibility that the patient accidentally over medicated. If the over medication is suspected, the pharmacist or medication bottle can provide information regarding when a prescription was filed, and for how many pills. The number of pills remaining in the bottle can indicate how many pills were taken since the prescription was filled and should correlate with the prescribed dose and frequency. Taking the medications to the hospital or showing them to the responder can help determine if overuse is the problem.

If the patient was injured by a fall, he should not be moved unless he is in a position that will cause him more harm. If the patient falls in the bathtub, be sure that his face is not submerged in water before calling for help, and turn off the water or drain the tub as warranted.

If the patient tries to get up, encourage him to remain still until he can be assessed by medical personnel. Do not force the patient to stay still by restraining him unless it is obvious that he can further injury himself by moving. If the patient is irrational, gently keep the patient in place by holding his hand and providing verbal support. If the patient is completely out of control or thrashing about, it may be necessary to let him go. Restraining a combative patient under any circumstance may lead to injury of the patient or caregiver. The ambulance response should be quick and the responders can decide the best way to control the patient if needed.

If an injury was sustained in a public setting, the responsible party and any witnesses should stay at the scene until the police have arrived. If a witness is unable or unwilling to stay, obtain her name and phone number. If a vehicle is involved and leaves the scene, try to remember or record the license plate number, color and make of the vehicle. Generally the person with the injured party is not focused on these details but a witness may take note.

Injury or crisis of any sort can result in physical and emotional shock to the victim. The caregiver should place a blanket or towel over the patient to help conserve body temperature and reduce shock. If a caregiver has no knowledge of emergency first aid, she should not feel responsible to provide direct care prior to emergency response. Classes that teach first aid and emergency care should be strongly considered by all caregivers.

13

DEATH AND DYING

Chronically ill patients usually have a primary doctor caring for them on a regular basis who is able to determine when their health is declining. The doctor may broach the subject with the patient and family, and explain what types of medication or treatments are available to prolong the patient's life and/or improve its quality. The doctor may discuss aggressive treatment plans, experimental drugs or surgery as appropriate. However, if the doctor feels that no further treatment is available or feasible, the issue of death may be addressed.

Each patient reacts differently when the doctor discusses the lack of further treatment. Patients who are familiar with death, sometimes because they cared for a spouse, child or friend during the dying process, or because they have strong religious beliefs, tend to accept the issue of impending death with less anxiety. Patients who have had little exposure to death, or who have never considered their own mortality, may have more difficulty. Afraid of a patient's reaction to the news, families sometimes request that patients are not told of a terminal diagnosis. If this is indicated, the patient will be told only what is necessary for his emotional and physical well being.

Whether aware of their condition or not, every patient deserves the opportunity to die with dignity, in a safe and comfortable environment. This can be done at home or in a hospice.

After a terminal diagnosis, referral to a home based or free standing hospice—a facility that provides care for terminally ill patients—may be made. Such facilities may have a religious affiliation or be part of a nursing home or hospital. The approach to care at a hospice is generally to keep the patient comfortable and provide emotional support.

If the patient chooses to enter such a facility, he should help choose the facility. The doctor, nurse or social worker, either at home or from the hospital, can assist with the admissions procedure. The institution will have its own admissions department for further information. The patient should be aware of any limit to the amount and type of personal belongings the hospice allows, as well as its visiting policy. Young children and pets are sometimes allowed to visit only at the discretion of the facility.

If the patient decides to continue his care at home without hospice involvement, a visiting nurse can be referred. The nurse can help institute a plan of care and be available for emotional support. The extent of involvement will be determined by the patient and family, who may wish to have limited nursing in order to care for the patient themselves during such a personal and emotional time, or vice versa. Nursing service that is refused or limited initially can be expanded at a later time if the patient's needs change.

When dying at home, the patient and/or caregiver needs to maintain frequent and candid communication with the doctor. Some doctors may offer their home phone numbers for easier access, or may make home visits to assess the dying patient.

Pain medications may be altered in dose or frequency to allow greater pain relief. Less emphasis may be placed on potential side effects of the medication and more on the patient's immediate needs. For this reason, the doctor may agree to discontinue any medications that cause uncomfortable side effects such as nausea, fatigue or sleeplessness.

Sometimes the patient or caregiver may choose to seek emergency medical intervention after previously deciding otherwise. If the patient begins to have frequent or severe complaints, or as death approaches, the family or patient may not wish to continue care at home. Interventions may become more complicated. The patient can require more care than the caregivers are physically or emotionally able to provide. Every effort should be made to hospitalize or place the patient in a health facility if no reasonable alternative exists.

At times, a person familiar with the patient's desire to die at home may intervene to help caregivers examine the factors that lead them to plan for death and dying at home. Frank discussion and honest response by the caregivers may lead them to reconsider staying at home or accept that more constant or intense medical treatment can be provided in an institution.

Plans for home care are just that, plans. They are not binding agreements, but attempts to meet the patient's immediate health care needs. Changes in plans, or reductions in caregivers' participation are not failures, but are an indication that the home care process is working in the patient's best interests.

COUNSELING

Pastoral counselors can be utilized by the patient and caregivers to sift through the emotional impact of death. They can help resolve any feelings of fear, despair or anxiety that arise. The patient's religious counselor may also provide comfort and meet his spiritual needs, especially if they have a long-standing relationship.

Patients need to be reassured that their needs and those of their caregivers will be met. It is not unusual for a patient to seek nursing home placement or hospitalization to spare the family the strain of care at home. The family should speak candidly to the patient regarding their own desire and ability to care for the patient. Avoiding the issue can lead to guilt and regrets when it is too late to reverse the decision.

As patients get older, they often feel that they are a burden to their families or worry that they have limited financial resources to obtain adequate home care. Many do not realize that their insurance might pay for home care or hospice services. A social worker may be able to help determine the patient's benefits, and put the patient's mind at ease.

Caregivers also need counseling. The emotional aspects of death and dying are tremendous. Many patients feel guilty that they did not identify signs of disease or complications, that they delayed health care or refused follow up treatment. The patient may be sad at not being present to witness family milestones. The patient and caregiver may also feel isolated and be uncomfortable discussing their roles. Formal support from professionals or support groups can help relieve some of the isolation, and a group approach by all family members can diffuse the responsibilities.

ADVANCED DIRECTIVES

The patient should have a health care directive so that his wishes regarding the extent of medical intervention are known. Often, family members may have different opinions regarding life support measures, so the directive is a valuable tool in uniting family members to seek the most appropriate patient care. The doctor's understanding of the patient's wishes may also be helpful and may prevent unnecessary intervention during a medical crisis.

When death occurs, all measures to resuscitate the patient will be made unless otherwise immediately indicated in an advance directive or living will. Therefore, all persons in the home should be aware of any such documents.

The patient may choose to be an organ donor if medical conditions warrant. The doctor can provide information regarding the feasibility of such a decision, and can assist the patient in completing correct releases. If the patient is an organ donor, the ambulance will need to be notified immediately after the patient's death to ensure proper arrangements.

DEATH

Deaths at home need to be reported to the police, who will dispatch an ambulance. If death was suspicious or unanticipated the police may investigate, or if the patient was not under recent doctor's care an autopsy may be performed.

Depending on state laws, death in the home might be pronounced by a coroner, a hospice nurse, an emergency medical worker or the police. The patient will be released to the funeral parlor from the home if an autopsy is not needed. Communicating the patient's religious affiliation, especially if it requires immediate burial, may speed the release process unless an investigation is necessary.

For patients who did not wish to have medical intervention, or if death had occurred hours before the patient was found and resuscitation would not have been productive, the ambulance company will follow its internal policy regarding patient care or lack thereof.

On rare occasions, family members feel that resuscitation should be performed on the patient regardless of the signs that death occurred long enough in the past to make revival impossible. Because of the finality of death and the intense emotions involved, every effort should be made to reassure this person that interventions would be futile.

There are as many signs of impending death as there are people that die. Patients may have changes in breathing, heart rate or blood pressure that can be observed by a nurse or doctor, who can then alert the family that death is near. At other times, patients simply go to sleep and do not wake up.

Muscles in the mouth, rectum and urinary tract often relax after or during death causing a release of body fluids. The caregiver and/or family members do not need to take action to clean the patient, but may choose to be involved for religious or emotional reasons. These preparations will be done by the funeral home prior to removing the patient from the home.

FUNERAL ARRANGEMENTS

Patients who are alert prior to death may want to participate in planning their visitation or funeral. This preparation can be done long before death becomes imminent or predictable. An advocate from a funeral home can assist the patient with planning, and the patient may even choose to pay for the arrangements prior to his death. Having a family member or advocate available during this planning will help facilitate the patient's plans so that details are not omitted. Often, the patient is reassured to know that his wishes will be carried out. This may be the patient's way of maintaining some control over an otherwise unpredictable event.

The patient may further choose to give away possessions and assets prior to her death so that she can be sure that those receiving them understand any special attachment she had to them. A mirror or scarf that may be discarded after death might have had significant meaning to the patient and the distribution of such items allows the patient to feel that the person receiving it will understand the sentimental or historical value.

A caregiver or advocate should supervise the distribution of belongings if not legally supported by a property will. This can reduce the appearance of opportunistic family and friends who may request specific items of the patient. If the patient is forgetful or confused, an attorney can help as an advocate for the patient.

Attempts to discourage visitors who may cause the patient anxiety, anger or who would not be welcome for personal reasons should be made when the patient's death is expected. If this is impossible, the visits should be supervised and a set period of time for the visits discussed. Family and caregivers can intervene if the visit becomes uncomfortable for the patient.

Patients may also make specific requests that flowers be omitted from services or that charitable contributions be made in their name. The funeral home makes arrangements for publication of obituaries and will provide this information to the media if indicated. Suggestions for charitable agencies may be made by the funeral director if requested. Many funeral homes have pre-printed envelopes available at visitations to facilitate contributions. The agency receiving the donations will provide a family member with a list of those who contributed so that the family can acknowledge the donation.

If a patient or family members request that donations be made in the patient's name to a scholarship, building or research fund, or that contributions be used for the welfare of their family, the funeral director will obtain specific details to receive the donations.

Flowers that are received at visitation are usually donated to local hospitals, nursing homes or the religious facilities after the services. Clothing, furniture or other possessions or collections belonging to the patient may be donated according to the patient's wishes.

Funeral directors will assist in the planning of all aspects of the visitation and burial proceedings including transportation, ceremonies, obtaining or re-opening burial plots, and the participation of religious personnel. If there are any specific songs, readings or persons that should be part of the ceremony, the funeral director can make the arrangements.

The funeral and visitation planning process begins with the family or advocate choosing a funeral home or facility. They must choose whether cremation, burial or entombment will be done. Coffins or other burial container will be chosen and clothing arranged. The funeral home will have a selection of coffins to look at, or the family may choose to have the director use his discretion. Clothing may be bought at the facility if not provided by the family.

A recent picture of the patient will assist the undertaker in preparing the body. Usual patient accessories such as glasses and dentures should be given along with the picture.

Family members may also wish to include favorite personal belongings, pictures or religious material in the casket to be buried with the patient. These items should be given to the funeral director with specific instruction that they are for burial.

Items that are with the patient during visitation such as glasses, jewelry or religious artifacts may be kept by the family. Funeral directors should offer these items to the family unless otherwise directed.

The duration of visitation will be set. The director may ask if a large number of people are expected so the most efficient arrangements can be made. The patient's church or synagogue will be notified by the funeral home to arrange for prayers at visitations and to make funeral plans. If the patient had a special relationship with a religious figure, that person will often attend. Many family members take more comfort when led in prayer by someone who knew the patient well and who is able to insert personal comments and emotion into the service. Transportation to and from funeral proceedings will be arranged and includes direction of traffic and funeral procession.

Pall bearers can be provided by family or are available as part of the funeral plan. The funeral director can offer suggestions for the person making the funeral plans regarding all aspects, including provision of seating at grave site ceremonies, and umbrellas and ground cover in the event of inclement weather.

The funeral director should have an effective and discrete plan for dealing with people who are emotionally upset or who may disturb the family. If the family anticipates that such a person may attend and cause a disturbance, the funeral director should be advised beforehand. He may ask for a description of the person or to be notified immediately when the person arrives. In the event that the person's death will evoke interest of the press, the director should be aware.

If hotel accommodations are needed, the director can recommend facilities. They can also recommend and arrange for post-funeral receptions.

Burial plots purchased prior to death or family plots will have a deed that must be provided. A fee to re-open a plot may be charged by the cemetery. Fees for funeral proceedings can be paid in installments and money may be set aside by the patient prior to death to cover these costs.

Burial markers may be arranged by the family independent of funeral proceedings. The site will be marked temporarily until a marker is obtained.

AFTER DEATH

When funeral proceedings are complete, the caregiver may need a grieving period before attending to the patient's environment. The removal of medical equipment from the home should be done as quickly as possible for insurance billing reasons. It may also help erase unsettling images of the patient when they were ill.

The need to return medical equipment may also lead into the disposal of the patient's belongings. When possible, all involved family should participate in the actual clearing out of the patient's living area, or should take part in making agreeable arrangements. By sifting through the patient's personal belongings, the family or caregivers may be comforted by the memories such items evoke.

If a paid caregiver was involved in the patient's care for a long period of time, or in close manner where a strong relationship developed, it would not be unusual to offer that person a token or reminder of the patient. Be sure that other family members who may not be aware of the extent of this relationship are told, so as to avoid confusion or accusations.

When a patient was living in a home in which children where raised, the distribution of content may become emotional and complicated. An advocate that can help confirm the patient's intentions may be helpful, or legal intervention required.

If there is not a rush to disperse the patient's belongings, doing so slowly, with careful consideration of what is to be kept and disposed of can reduce regrets later. It may be difficult or impossible to retrieve an item that is later thought to be valuable or nostalgic. If the home's contents must be disposed of immediately so that the home can be sold or re-arranged, try to store possessions for later examination. A company can be hired that will remove and dispose of the house or apartment contents. Furniture and other household items can be donated to charity, or catalogued for sale by professional estate sale services. Generally, the family can describe specific items to be set aside or stored, otherwise the contents are disposed of according to company policy. If making this arrangement from a distance and certain possessions are to be saved, be sure that a reputable company is used to prevent theft.

If the patient has financial obligations that must be taken care of by the sale of the home or possessions, an attorney should be contacted to make these arrangements.

At times, the mail will still arrive addressed to the patient. Utility companies should be contacted to turn off gas and electric so that billing stops. The post office should be notified to arrange the forwarding of the patient's mail as needed.

GRIEVING

When patients no longer require care at home because of death or long-term placement, the caregivers may find themselves experiencing grief. A variety of resources including books and support groups deal with the emotional aspects of death and dying, and they may help the caregiver identify specific emotions and begin the healing process. If the caregiver begins to feel despair or depression, professional intervention may be needed.

Support groups to which the caregiver may have belonged, or hospice agencies, often provide follow-up contact for caregivers. The ability to openly discuss feelings about the patient with someone who knew the patient, and the degree of care and involvement by the caregiver, may help validate the caregiver's emotions.

When the patient is an elderly parent, the support given to the caregiver at the time of the patient's death may unfortunately be limited, especially if the illness was prolonged. Family and friends may offer sympathy that is inappropriate if they are not aware of the extent of the caregiver's involvement.

The caregiver must know in her heart that she was an essential factor and critical element in maintaining the patient's dignity and medical well-being while helping with the patient's care at home. The decision to provide mental, physical and spiritual support for any patient at home is a reflection of selfless giving and commitment to that patient.

14

MAKING CARING EASIER

O rganizing a patient's care and establishing routines can make home care work better. The first step is to determine who will be calling the shots. In many cases, an adult child is the primary decision maker for the patient, or is largely influential in the patient's care. When possible, decision making should be shared by all family members. However, if there is only one responsible person, input from the doctor, clergy member, visiting nurse, friends and any knowledgeable resources can be helpful.

CHOOSING AN ADVOCATE

If choosing one family member as an advocate is not possible, or if opinions among family members regarding care differ, a third party may need to be involved. The use of an advocate for the patient, who will not be directly involved in care, may be done informally among family members and is sometimes effective in changing the view of family members whose ideas conflict.

In this case it is even more important that the patient be involved in any decisions so that her wishes are clearly stated. Doctors, clergy and close friends may be able to provide testimony to a patient's wishes if the patient is no longer able to voice them.

An attorney versed in elder law can provide a clear understanding of the financial and legal responsibilities that an advocate needs to consider. Power of attorney may be assigned, financial accounts transferred and personal belongings properly accounted for or dispersed. A candid discussion with the patient is best done before the need arises so the patient has full awareness and agreement as well as input regarding all decisions. The patient may need to sign legal papers transferring rights and, therefore, should be fully alert and understand all the proceedings. It is helpful to have the patient's mail forwarded to the primary caregiver's residence, to avoid misplacing bills or other important communication.

MONITORING THE PATIENT'S CONDITION

Having realistic expectations regarding a patient's potential for improvement or eventual death can make caring for that patient at home more manageable and less stressful. Patients who are discharged from the hospital after acute illness or surgery generally will need 6 to 8 weeks to start to feel as though they are getting "back to normal."

Improvement in the patient's status should be measured week to week instead of daily. Focus should be placed on what the patient can do, and the patient should be encouraged to be as independent as possible and participate in care and the planning of care when able.

The patient may have good days and bad days, which can prove frustrating to the caregiver. The issue of confusion or forgetfulness can be especially difficult if the patient has times when she is fully aware. The caregiver may have hopes that the improvement will persist, but when the patient resorts back to forgetfulness, the caregiver must respond accordingly. Attempts to anticipate periods of awareness and when they will end are almost impossible. The caregiver is offered a glimmer of hope that the patient is improving and when it is gone, may be left feeling that somehow he could have prolonged or reversed it altogether.

If the caregiver is informed about the disease process as well as about the patient's potential quality of life and life expectancy, the caregiver can develop a realistic understanding and acceptance of the patient's physical, emotional and mental states. To obtain this information, the caregiver must ask health care providers direct questions in order to receive direct and honest answers.

It is not uncommon for a patient to verbalize feelings that they are not going to live much longer. Some patients give up hope, and some look forward to death to relieve them of pain or the inability to accept their change in physical status or dependence on others. Though sometimes difficult for a caregiver to accept, these feelings should be discussed with the patient. Doctors, nurses, clergy, family or friends that are comfortable with this discussion should be contacted so the patient can be offered the opportunity to verbalize her feelings.

If the patient appears obsessed with dying, or verbalizes despair that death is not coming fast enough, she needs intervention from a mental health professional. Emergency intervention is available via telephone. Crisis intervention teams can assess the patient's potential to hurt herself and will dispatch emergency help accordingly. Patients in this state of mind should never be left alone, and medications or weapons that the patient may access should be removed from the environment.

A patient's wishes regarding the extent of medical treatment that they desire should be discussed and documented according to legal standards. Once this is done, the patient may be reassured that their desires will be respected and can change their emotional focus to enjoying the time that remains.

The patient's ability to understand and desire to know the diagnosis may be discussed by the doctor and family before giving the patient any information. It is not unusual for patients to be unaware that they have a terminal illness. However, any caregivers must know that the patient is unaware of the diagnosis so that they don't provide information inadvertently.

At times, especially if care is provided by a number of doctors, it may be unclear whether the patient is aware or of her medical status. A visiting nurse may ask the patient if she was diagnosed with cancer or other illness. If the patient answers, "No," it can be assumed that she is not aware.

The family may disagree on the amount of information that a patient needs to know. For example, one member may refer to the patient's illness, and another may deny that the patient is sick. This is a confusing situation for all involved and may lead to many conflicts. A family discussion, regarding how much information the patient needs to know or would want to know, must be had.

Patients with terminal illnesses, or those who are dying as a natural result of the aging process, often are intuitive regarding impending death. They may openly refer to the near future and that they won't be present for it. Caregivers who are comfortable discussing these feelings should explore them with the patient or call in a priest or professional to offer support.

THE DIFFICULTIES OF CAREGIVING

Old Habits Die Hard

Caregivers need to remember that the patient may not easily change her old habits or may not be able to understand restrictions. Cigarette and alcohol use pose a health and safety hazard, but the doctor may okay limited and supervised use. Consideration of these habits is especially important when the patient will be residing with the caregiver. The comfort and safety of others who are already living in the residence needs to be considered.

Realistic Expectations

Caregivers need to be realistic about their ability to participate, both physically and emotionally, in patient care. The emotional response to caring for a sick or elderly parent can be overwhelming. The complicated role changes can be frustrating and anxiety provoking, especially when money, time, distance and commitments to other family members are involved. It can be stressful when no other support is available to give the caregiver relief.

Caregivers may find that they are performing tasks for their parents that they find embarrassing, such as bathing or feeding, or distasteful, such as changing diapers or cleaning up vomit. By attending support groups, the caregiver may be able to network with other informal caregivers who can perform some of these tasks for them, offer coping mechanisms, or simply agree that they find the care beyond their realm too.

Seeking Support

Support groups can put the caregiver in touch with others who are in similar situations and allow sharing of ideas and emotions. Participation at meetings is encouraged but not mandatory, so a caregiver can attend just to listen. At times the caregiver can benefit from just getting out of the home for a period of time, but may feel that she is not justified in doing so without a purpose. Support groups can provide this purpose.

By attending these meetings, the caregiver can obtain ideas for making care more effective. Listening to others describe situations similar to those that the caregiver is experiencing can often reduce fear, anxiety and feelings of isolation. Knowing that others get angry, tired and frustrated can help a caregiver acknowledge her own feelings. Validating that she is caring for the patient in much the same way as others do can reassure her that she is doing all that can be done.

Computers are valuable tools. The internet offers many web sites with valuable information regarding disease processes and current treatments as well as support groups. Be aware, however, that the vast amount of information available on the internet comes with no guarantee regarding its source, validity or credentials.

Delegating Care

Sometimes, one family member will appear to the rest of the family to be the best choice for providing care. This situation arises most often with the child that lives closest, was favored by the parent, does not have a spouse or children, or has experience with health and medicine. Delegating responsibility or scheduling a rotation of caregivers can help reduce this pressure.

The primary caregiver can assign each participating family member a task, such as taking the patient to the doctor or on outings, paying bills, or providing groceries and/or meals. Planning to have family members take over for a day or weekend can help the primary caregiver cope with the responsibility and provide some time for rest. For this reason, all potential caregivers should be given routine accounts of the patient's status changes and treatments. If this is done, having another family member relieve the primary caregiver for a period of time is less threatening and more easily facilitated. For family that excuse themselves because they feel that they lack the knowledge for care, offer to have them come for a day prior to their scheduled time to be taught patient care.

If family members are unable or unwilling to assist in care, they can be asked for financial assistance to hire additional care when needed. Sometimes the family will be more willing to participate in patient care when presented with the cost of hired care.

Patients may split their living time between different homes. As long as each place is equipped to meet the patient's needs with caregivers and proper environment, the patient and primary caregivers may benefit from such an arrangement. This plan must be carefully evaluated if the patient is forgetful or confused because the patient may need the continuity of familiar settings in order to function best.

Time Off

Time away from the patient is important for any caregiver who provides constant patient care. This allows the caregiver to have some physical and emotional rest. Being constantly responsible for the care of another person is fatiguing and when it is a loved one, feelings of guilt, sadness and indecision may occur. Home care aids or private nurses can be hired for short term care such as a weekend. Agencies will discuss patient needs with the caregiver prior to assignment so that the aid or nurse will be able to provide all treatments and follow regimes.

All caregivers need emotional and physical support. Professional staff have other members of the team and agency who can offer advice or counseling as needed when caring for a particular patient becomes complex or overwhelming. However, informal caregivers may be isolated by the lack of time off and burdened by the responsibility of care. The patient's needs are often put first, with the caregiver forgoing his or her own medical or social commitments in order to provide the care. The role reversal faced by a child caring for a parent may be particularly stressful. As often as possible, in any way available, a caregiver should seek the guidance and support of formal and informal resources.

15

ALTERNATIVES TO HOME CARE

OUTPATIENT CLINICS

Outpatient rehabilitation may be hospital based or performed at free-standing facilities. Concentrated attention is focused on the patient's affected body parts or systems with an assessment of the patient's rehabilitation potential. A doctor must make the referral for outpatient therapy, and will order specific levels or types of activity that should be attained or avoided.

Outpatient programs may be able to provide certain types of treatment, such as hydro-therapy, that require large pieces of equipment that are not available in the home. Patients must be able to get to the facility, sometimes as often as five times a week. Transportation might be arranged or provided by the facility.

Some patients continue to work or maintain their social obligations, and they schedule their outpatient therapy accordingly. While the patient is receiving outpatient rehabilitation, the nurse may still visit the home to provide education and care.

LONG TERM CARE FACILITIES

Long term health care facilities provide ongoing medical intervention 24 hours a day. The patient, caregiver or doctor may choose such a facility if the patient's needs are related to an unstable medical condition that responds predictably to interventions when the need arises, or is frequently unstable but not life threatening. This patient would not need hospital care, but does require constant medical intervention.

Long term care may also be considered when patient care becomes complicated, frequent or intense, and caregivers are no longer able to devote the time or skills required.

Some long term facilities have short term rehabilitation divisions that attempt to restore the patient to some level of independence. If successful, the patient may be discharged to the home with adequate support from formal and informal caregivers. If the patient is unable to be rehabilitated, he is transferred to the long term care division.

The decision to place a patient in a long term facility and its admissions process requires examining the patient's acceptance and understanding of placement, the family's or advocate's participation in the decision, and a doctor's referral. Insurance information and an examination of the patient's assets will determine the fee structure. The facility can advise of their specific admissions criteria, how all aspects can be met including medical information and assessment of the patient's need for care. Counseling of patient and family can assist in meeting the emotional needs that arise when making the decision to place the patient in such a facility.

RETIREMENT COMMUNITIES

Retirement communities, also called assisted living communities, are organized environments for older people. Admission is elective and lifestyle is independent. The patient should be in generally stable health and able to meet his or her own needs for grooming, cooking and medical treatments. Many of these settings provide organized trips for social events and shopping.

Generally, the patient will be responsible for managing his finances. However, some community settings have the patient's monthly stipend sent directly to them to pay the patient's rent and utilities. The balance is then given to the patient. This structuring allows for the financial success of the community. However, the patient should be aware of these policies prior to accepting living arrangements.

Homes within a retirement community can be purchased or rented. Some offer shared living in townhouses or apartment buildings. Some institution-type settings contain infirmaries that can care for patients as they recover from illness or surgery. Plan to meet with the director of any institution prior to making any decisions to arrange a tour and have questions answered. Also, plan to meet and speak to some current residents to get the best sense of how the community functions. An attorney who practices elder law can assist a patient when exploring retirement communities. This type of advocacy can aid the patient in choosing the arrangement that meets his or her financial needs and protects their assets.

Medical insurance does not cover retirement community living, but may allow for home health care within the patient's home in such a setting.

WOUND CARE

Wound care centers are a more recent alternative to the ongoing needs of patients with chronic or recurring skin breakdown. Actual wound care and patient instruction in self care is done by the staff.

A patient may need to visit every day until care can be taught. On the other hand, frequency of visits may be increased if the patient is unable to learn care or the wound site is not accessible to them.

Wound care centers may also provide aggressive or experimental treatments, but the patient should check if her insurance will cover it.

The doctor who plans the patient's wound care is generally employed by the center and will consult the patient's primary doctor as needed. The patient may also have intermittent care by a visiting nurse who will supervise the patient's ability to carry out wound treatment at home. The visiting nurse will communicate any concerns to the center's staff and/or doctor.

Transportation may be provided or arranged by the center. Fees for transportation can be incorporated into treatment billing. The insurance may not cover transportation or wound care center services unless state certifications for the center are maintained.

OUTPATIENT DAY CARE

Outpatient day care centers are an alternative to standard home care. These types of programs generally do not require a doctor's order for admittance, but the doctor may need to provide information about the patient's status prior to admission.

Outpatient programs provide socialization, structured events, and meals for the patients. The staff usually consists of nurses, a social worker, a service coordinator, and admissions and ancillary staff.

Patients may receive medications, including injections of insulin, and special diet requirements can be observed. Patients' blood pressure and other vital functions can be assessed on a regular interval and the results can be called in to the doctor if untypical for the patient.

Outpatient programs may be located at local senior citizen homes, adjacent to nursing homes or hospitals, or may be free standing. Many programs provide transportation to and from the site, with assistance in and out of the building.

Day programs are a reasonable alternative to traditional home care, and they have the added benefit of allowing the patient to get out of her home environment and be around others.

Payment for these services may be arranged by the day, week, or month depending on agency policy.

Skilled home nursing visits may be coordinated with outpatient care. Some patients may attend outpatient care three days a week and have nursing visits on the other days if needed for daily injections or wound care.

Insurance coverage varies, and may not be available at all. Some programs are subsidized by local, state or federal grants, so discuss payment options with the admissions coordinator before making any commitments.

Information regarding outpatient services may be obtained by word of mouth, ads in newspapers or magazines, the yellow pages, hospital social service offices, doctors, home care agencies or local offices of the aging.

HOSPICE CARE

Hospice is a service that provides care for patients with a terminal diagnosis. Traditional hospice programs require that the patient be admitted for care only after the doctor provides documentation that the patient has six months or less to live, is aware of the diagnosis and life expectancy, and has agreed not to seek emergency services in the event of a decline in their physical status. The patient must also agree not to seek treatment that will prolong their life expectancy such as chemotherapy or radiation.

A patient who agrees to hospice care is at liberty to revoke that decision, but insurance coverage varies regarding the patient's decision to resume hospice care at a later date. For example, a patient with a terminal cancer diagnosis may decide to go off of hospice care if a new procedure or medication becomes available that may prolong her life. If she tries the new treatment and it is not effective, the insurance company may refuse to pay for her to go back on hospice. Some insurance companies have a waiting period before hospice can be resumed, and others may pay for hospice care only for a specific period of time.

Hospice provide services not usually offered by traditional home care, such as religious counseling, respite care (giving the patient's personal caregiver time off from patient care with the use of trained hospice volunteers), and 24-hour nursing availability for emergency intervention. By contrast, a home care agency generally has a nurse available by phone 24 hours-a-day who will recommend transport to an emergency facility as needed, or will arrange for the patient to be seen on the following work day.

Neither hospice nor home care agencies are able to provide for emergency care in the home. A hospice approach would be to visit and assess the extent of injury or change in condition, and call the doctor for orders. If a hospice patient's medical condition begins to decline, the nurse will support the personal caregivers through the decline and eventual death of the patient at home. This is what the hospice philosophy is based on.

Home care nurses will advise via phone to seek emergency room service for medical emergency and arrange ambulance service for the patient if an injury occurs at home. In the event of a change in physical status that does not require emergency intervention, a nurse may make an additional unscheduled nursing visit during scheduled office hours. This may occur if a patient has a wound that appears or reopens, or if the patient has a feeding or drainage tube that becomes dislodged. The nurse can assess the situation and act on it with the supplies that are available in the home.

Hospice insurance benefits may also include payment for medications and supplies not usually covered by standard insurance, and may provide for unlimited nursing and ancillary service visits.

Free-standing hospices do exist and some religious orders provide hospice type services for the terminal ill.

There are many disease processes besides cancer that are appropriate for hospice referral. An honest discussion with the primary doctor regarding the patient's medical status and life expectancy, and an assessment of the patient's needs—both physical and emotional—can aid the caregiver when considering hospice.

NURSING HOME

If patient care at home becomes impossible for the caregiver or fails to adequately meet the patient's needs, permanent placements in a long term care facility may be indicated. Placement in such a facility should be discussed with the patient and doctor, as well as other family members.

If placement is strongly opposed by the patient, arrangements for continuous care by paid professionals at home may need to be arranged. The cost of such care may be prohibitive, but obtaining costs and allowing the patient to clearly see that every attempt is being made to keep the patient home may reduce the patient's resistance. Supplementing informal caregivers with professional assistance may also be an alternative.

If the only possible solution becomes placement, the patient should be involved in choosing the institution. The level of care that the patient needs will be assessed by a specially trained nurse and supported by a doctor's medical documentation. Financial and insurance information will also need to be provided.

When choosing a facility, consideration may be given to religious affiliation, location of facility in relation to family members, and the provision of special services such as day trips for socialization or special disease-specific needs.

If the patient will never be returning home, assist them in the choosing personal items to bring with them.

If the institution allows, and the patient is physically able, they may be taken out for holidays or other celebrations.

Facilities vary in the levels of skilled medical care available on site and levels of nursing care that they provide. The patient's level of independence will be considered when placing them on a unit in the institution.

The decision to place a patient in a long term care facility can be agonizing for the family regardless of the patients acceptance or lack of it. By keeping in mind that this is the best alternative for the patient, the family may be relieved of some of the emotional conflict.

The ability to visit a facility at any time of day may be a consideration when making a choice of institution but the primary factor in this decision should be the ability of the institution to meet the patients needs. Before placement, the family should be offered a tour so that they can see the staff at work and observe the interactions with patients. If an institution provides a living arrangement that is in keeping with the patients style of living, ethnic and religious concerns, the transition may be easier.

Allowing a period of adjustment for the family and patient can ease uncertainty. Candid discussion with family of other residents or with the residents themselves can also help.

Communicating a patient's specific dietary likes, dislikes or daily routines, and any ways that the caregiver has found most effective or comforting in approaching the patient, can help the nursing home staff make the adjustment easier. Ask the charge nurse or administrator if family participation in care is allowed or encouraged. The ability to continue to contribute to a patient's care may be comforting to the family.

On occasion, patients' families choose to remove them from a facility when or if care at home becomes feasible. This may be due to a positive change in the patient's status or the fact that adequate support systems have been obtained.

If the original plan before admission was to eventually take the patient back home or install them in a different setting, choice of institution may be different than that for a permanent admission.

Insurance coverage may have restrictions for patients who are removed from an extended care facility. There may be a final determination that coverage will not be allowable for admission at a later date or the period that the patient was in the facility may not be paid for or done so with limitations.

By fully understanding an insurance policy's allowances and restrictions, as well as coverage for unusual situations, costly interventions may be avoided.

A case manager may be assigned to provide a contact person who can aid on an individual basis. The facility should also have a social worker on premises who can advise current trends in coverage.

At any time, if a concern arises that the level of care does not meet the caregiver's or patient's needs, it must be discussed with the administrator immediately. All communication in this situation should be documented regarding time, date and person with whom it was discussed, and any follow up plan with date expected to rectify situation. By doing this, supporting documentation can be provided to the insurance company if a patient is removed because the facility does not meet their needs. Of course, the needs must pertain to the maintenance of a patient's health and the delivery of treatments. Complaints regarding television programming or hair styles would not be considered high priority.

Social workers can supply a list of health care facilities and detail the admission criteria, costs, acceptance of insurance and levels of care provided.

16

PROFESSIONAL CARE PROVIDERS

T he knowledge and experience of a professional staff serves to enhance patient care at home. By working together as a team, each discipline focuses on meeting specific patient needs through its care and teaching.

The primary informal caregiver who is aware of the goals and expectations of each home care service may be able to avoid the confusion that can result from having many people involved.

What follows is a description of the general roles and services of each formal caregiver.

FOR ALL HOME CARE PROVIDERS

- Name, agency and phone number, position, expected frequency of visits per week, expected length of each visit, expected weeks of care.
- How the provider's service is being paid for.
- What they expect to provide for the patient.
- Where the patient should be located for visits and how they should be dressed. Valuable time is wasted when a home care visit is scheduled for a specific time and the patient is eating a meal or sleeping. Patients who require wound care may be directed to stay in bed until the nurse arrives. A therapist may want to see a patient on the second floor of a home if working on stair climbing. A patient who will be receiving a bath from a home health aid need not be dressed in street clothes for the visit. Of course, there are exceptions when a patient must use the bathroom while the therapist visits, or feels more comfortable in street clothes when the aid arrives. Explaining any of the patient's concerns at the onset of treatment will allow the care provider to adjust the schedule accordingly.

- If a primary therapist, nurse or aid is aware that they will be unable to attend the patient because of a scheduled absence from work, the name of the replacement and anticipated change in time of schedule should be provided to the patient or caregiver. Agencies make all attempts to schedule replacements in the same time frame and with a consistent service provider.

- Any information the caregiver does not want the patient to know, such as diagnosis (with the approval and knowledge of the doctor), payment/cost of services, or the possibility of re-hospitalization if scheduled.

- Times of day during which the patient is more alert, energetic or responds better to direction. Scheduled nap times that leave the patient feeling better should not be interrupted unless necessary to deliver medications or timed treatments.

- Always remember that, despite the fact the providers are assisting the patient, they are in the patient's home and should be respectful of the surroundings. Properly wiping their feet, being aware of fragile items and knocking on closed doors before opening them are just some of the basic good manners that can be overlooked by providers. If the patient's privacy or basic rights as a human being are ever not being considered, ask that caregiver to leave.

- If a caregiver is particularly helpful or involved, a note to the director of the agency praising their work is an easy and positive action. Home health care agencies are unable to constantly be aware of the degree or level of care provided by their employees. Comments from those who witness the hands-on care provided are a valuable resource and quality assurance tool.

THE DOCTOR

Patients generally have a primary physician that cares for their needs on a regular basis and is familiar with the patient's medical and personal concerns. The following is a list of points to consider in order to get the most appropriate care for the patient by the doctor.

- The doctor's credentials in his or her field, certifications and associations with medical groups and teaching facilities.

- Billing structure. Does the doctor request payment up front or bill the insurance for the patient? Is the doctor willing to accept partial payment or installments for fees? And what are the overall costs of services?

- Does the doctor participate in the patient's insurance plan? A doctor who is a participating provider in a health plan is obligated to accept the set rate from the insurance company for the approved and necessary exam or procedure. The patient is obligated to pay their co-payment *only*.

- Affiliation. Is the doctor associated with a group of doctors, and if so, is the patient familiar and comfortable with all participating doctors?

- Availability to make home visits to the patient, and any extra fees generated by a home visit. What is the doctor's familiarity with the range of services available at home, and his comfort in using them?

- Affiliation with the hospital of the patient's choice, and with major medical centers providing high tech surgery or experimental treatment.

- Availability of medical testing and laboratory facilities in the doctor's office or medical building.

- Accessibility of the doctor's office and adequate parking. This is especially important for patients with limited activity tolerance, patients who are driving themselves to appointments, or those who are using oxygen systems when making visits. If there are many stairs to climb or distant parking, visits may be difficult.

- What is the doctor's understanding of the patient's philosophy and wishes regarding the aggressiveness of medical intervention they may need or desire, and honesty with the patient regarding alternatives to, and expected outcomes of treatment?

- Hours that the doctor is available for visits so coordination of the personal caregiver's time may be considered.

- What is the doctor's knowledge of the patient as person, including work, family and personal history and how this impacts the patient's ability to access health care?

- The doctor should encourage the patient's involvement in his or her own care and suggest that the patient come to visits with a list of questions so that specific concerns about treatment or health complaints get covered.

PHYSICAL, OCCUPATIONAL AND SPEECH THERAPISTS

- The tentative plan for care, which will be altered according to the patient's response to interventions, treatments and as healing occurs.

- Ask whether pain medications should be given at a specific time prior to the therapist's visit. Medications that result in lethargy or confusion will adversely affect the therapy session. Conversely, if pain leaves the patient less able to perform therapy, it may need to be taken an hour before the visit to allow maximum participation by the patient.

- Have the proper equipment in the location along with any written information that the therapist has given in the past. Most patients will be provided with some degree of written home exercises based on their abilities, support and environment that they can practice in-between therapist visits and will continue after discharge from therapy.

- Ask if exercises can be taught to all caregivers involved, then make sure that the caregivers are present either as a group or scheduled to visit at the same time as the therapist. If a nurse is involved in care, the arrangement to coordinate home health aid hours with therapy visits can be done through the agency. It may not be necessary to have the caregiver present for each visit, only as many as the therapist feels will accomplish teaching.

- Tell the therapist if the patient has had a particularly good or poor response to the interventions since the last visit. This allows the therapist to re-arrange treatment if necessary.

- Let the therapist know if the patient has any appointments scheduled. Therapy can then focus on activities that the patient must perform to get to their appointment, including stair climbing, irregular surface walking or getting in and out of the car.

- If the therapist suggests equipment, ask who will be providing it, what it will cost, rental vs. purchase options, and if it needs to be installed, who will be doing that

SOCIAL WORKER

- When the social worker calls to make an appointment, ask what insurance, personal or financial documents they will need to see. The social worker may make an initial visit to determine the patient's needs before offering possible interventions. At that point, proper supporting documentation may be needed.

- Ask the social worker about experiences with other patients in similar situations, and how the interventions were discussed with patients, resistant family members and what were the outcomes of the interventions.

- Take all written information offered by the social worker, especially related to local or community resources. The contacts may be needed at a later date when a social worker may not be involved.

- Ask all questions regarding insurance coverage, even those that do not relate to the patient at the present time, because they may be relevant later. Over the long term, the patient may require equipment or services that may be accessed sooner if insurance coverage is fully understood.

- Ask if there are any current laws or practices being considered that may impact the patient's care or entitlements.

- Ask if you can contact the social worker after the patient is discharged from home care for additional resource information.

- Ask for phone numbers of medical suppliers that may carry products particularly helpful to the patient.

HOME HEALTH AID

- Obtain a written schedule of the times the aid is scheduled to visit so the schedule of other caregivers can be arranged.

- Plan for the primary caregiver to take a break from patient care when the aid visits. This is a good time for the caregiver to go for a walk, take a nap, go to the grocery store or perform any of the chores that can't be done if the patient needs constant supervision and intervention.

- The home health aid should be introduced to the patient and caregiver by the agency supervisor or representative. This joint visit should include an observation by the supervisor of how the aid interacts with the patient and how care should best be provided. Discuss with the aid and supervisor at the initial visit any suggested approaches to the patient or concerns of the patient's. Establishing a routine early in care provides the most efficient care.

- The aid is the person who will assist with the intimate details of bathing and dressing the patient, and a professional approach is always expected. If personality clashes arise or the care becomes questionable, contact the agency at once for a replacement or re-supervision of the aid. Many patients become afraid that if they complain, the aid will somehow retaliate. Patients, especially those that live alone or who are fragile, may accept inferior quality of care or be wary of voicing opinions or preferences because they feel defenseless. Others may feel grateful that they are getting any help at all regardless of quality.

- Remember that the aid is assigned her patients and is not directly involved in determining the frequency or length of visits.

- Direct any concerns or questions to the primary nurse or home health aid supervisor. The aid can notify her supervisor if the patients level of dependence increases and care takes longer than the time allotted.

NURSES

- Ask the nurse to write down blood pressure or temperature results.

- Ask the nurse to call the pharmacy for prescription refills if the patient has trouble doing so.

- If overseeing care from a distance, ask the nurse to call you with the findings of each visit and the plan for the next one.

- Request all the information that is available from the nurse regarding diet, medications, disease process and treatments.

- Ask for specific times for each medication administration and when it should be taken in relation to meals.

- Discuss discharge plans for the patient. Ask any questions you may have about care for the future and the likely alternatives.

- Ask for examples of patients that the nurse has known with similar diseases, symptoms or treatment plans. Sometimes, just knowing that there are situations like your own relieves some anxiety.

MEDICAL EQUIPMENT

- Get all phone numbers and names of contact people, including after hour services.

- Find out what the billing date is for rental equipment. When it is no longer needed, it may be returned before the start of the new cycle.

- Ask for policies on returning partially used boxes of supplies. Some companies have a donation program to a hospice or other non-profit agency.

- If you have a hospital bed or other large piece of equipment delivered, let the supplier know prior to deliver if the patient's bed or other furniture must be moved or rearranged by them. This allows for scheduling of proper personnel and allowances for the time involved.

17

GLOSSARY

T he definitions provided are for use within the context of this book. Many of the words are defined as they relate to an assessment of the patient and are symptoms and tools for documentation purposes. Many diseases, diagnosis and symptoms vary in occurrence and severity.

activities of daily living (ADL): ADL refers to the patient's ability to participate in or provide their own bathing, mouth care, dressing, toileting, meal preparation, and care of the home. Levels of ADL's vary throughout active illness and recovery, and assessment of baseline needs helps when planning care.

activity tolerance: Amount or frequency of mobility, transfers and position change that a patient can perform without excess fatigue.

acute illness: Period of a disease or series of symptoms requiring rapid intervention.

adaptive device: Item used to make a specific task or action easier.

adult protective: Agency involved on patient's behalf when resources are inadequate or non-existent to meet an adult's needs. May relate to medical, social, economic or environmental concerns.

advanced directive: Collective term to define a patient's wishes regarding medical intervention. This is a legal format which must be signed, dated and witnessed. The directive must be executed in the state in which it will be carried out, though laws and accepted practices may vary.

advocate: Person who acts on behalf the patient in their best interest. An advocate may be chosen by the patient or may be self appointed to support the patient's wishes or help direct or manage their care.

ambulate: To move or walk about.

ambulette: A van-like vehicle equipped to transport patients who have physical disabilities or limitations.

ancillary services: Services beyond nursing care including physical therapy, occupational therapy, home health aid and social worker.

antibiotic: Medication given to inhibit bacterial growth.

apathetic: Lack of in interest or emotion.

assessment: Examination of the patient—medical, environmental and social.

bacteria: Microorganisms that can cause disease or infection.

bedpan: Small, flat metal or plastic device that is placed under a patient as a receptacle for urine or/and stool. After use it is emptied, cleaned and can be re-used.

blood thinners: Type of medication that delays blood clotting, may cause increased potential for bleeding and bruising.

brand name: Manufacturer-specific medication name, usually shorter and easier to pronounce.

cardiopulmonary: Relating to the heart and lungs.

cardio-pulmonary resuscitation (CPR): Technique used to attempt to restore heart and/or lung function when cardiac or respiratory arrest occur.

caregiver: Person who is involved in delivery of or overseeing patient care. A "formal" caregiver is professionally trained, either paid or volunteer, to provide a particular service. An "informal" caregiver may be a family member or friend

catheter: Hollow tube that drains fluid from a cavity or body area. Foley catheter is a brand name and most often is used for urine drainage.

central venous catheter: An intravenous device threaded directly into a large vessel leading to the heart. It is inserted using sterile technique.

chemotherapy: Delivery of medication to inhibit or reduce the growth of cancerous cells.

choking: Obstruction of the air pipe resulting in reduced air flow. Needs immediate intervention that can be provided by the Heimlich maneuver.

chronic illness: Period of disease with more predictable and persistent symptoms.

circulation: Path the blood flow takes as it travels through the body.

clammy: When skin becomes damp and cold. May occur as a symptom of disease or as a reaction to medication.

colostomy: A surgical opening from the colon to the outside of the body for excretion to take place. May be permanent related to disease or temporary to allow a part of the intestines to rest or heal.

comatose: An extended state of unconsciousness.

commode: Chair-like portable toilet.

compress: Use of a washcloth or other soft cloth to apply heat or cold to a body part.

congestive heart failure (CHF): Disease or acute symptom rendering the heart unable to contract enough to pump all of the blood out of the heart.

contamination: Introduction of an organism that can cause infection.

constipation: Difficult or infrequent passage of stool.

co-payment: Dollar amount that the patient is required to pay a provider under the insurance plan. May be a pre-determined fee or a percentage of the total bill.

crisis: A sudden change for the worse during an illness.

cyanotic: Bluish discoloration of lips or skin caused by lack of oxygen.

defecate: The act of passing stools/feces from the bowels.

dehydration: Lack of sufficient fluid intake or within the body to maintain normal cell function.

dependent: Needing another to meet one's needs. May also be used to describe the position of a body part that is not supported e.g., legs that are not elevated when a patient is sitting are described as dependent.

diagnosis: Determination of the cause or nature of an illness.

diarrhea: Frequent, loose stools beyond the patient's normal bowel pattern.

dilate: When a structure expands beyond its natural dimensions.

discharge: When treatment ends, either in a facility or in the home. Is also used to describe drainage from a mucous membrane.

discharge planner: The person responsible for identifying a patient's post-hospital or -facility needs and implementing a plan with the doctor to meet those needs.

discharge summary: A written report highlighting events of hospital stay and plans for post hospital or facility care.

disposable: Meant to be thrown away after use.

diuretic: Type of medication that increases the amount of urine produced.

double bag: A technique of putting one bag of garbage or waste inside another to help reduce potential for contamination.

drainage: Fluids that are produced as waste from a wound or body cavity.

durable medical equipment (DME): General term that includes all equipment and supplies used by the patient at home.

edema: General or local swelling resulting from excess amount of tissue fluid.

elder law: Portions of laws relating specifically to the aging person. Attorneys may advertise as specialists in elder-law or offer seminars regarding the rights and options available.

electrolyte: Substances necessary to maintain cell and therefore body function. e.g. potassium and chloride.

endurance: Patients capacity for activity.

enema: Introduction of water or prescribed fluid into the rectum via a tube to stimulate bowel evacuation.

enteral: Feedings delivered directly into the digestive tract.

exacerbate: To make worse or more severe.

excoriate: To wear away the skin.

feces: Solid waste produced as by-product of the digestive process; stool.

feeding tube: A hollow tube inserted into a specific area of the gastrointestinal tract to facilitate feeding.

feeding syringe: A 60cc syringe structured with a wider opening than usual to allow delivery of liquid feeding into a feeding tube.

flow rate: The prescribed drops per minute for IV or enteral feedings, or liters per minute (lpm) for oxygen delivery.

friction: Rubbing of one surface against another.

gastrointestinal (GI): Relating to the digestive and intestinal systems.

generic: Drug classification, opposite of brand name; available for each manufacturer.

genitourinary (GU): Related to the genital and urinary systems.

guarding: The reflexive act by the patient of protecting a painful site.

halo vision: A symptom described as seeing a haze or blur around an object in the visual field that itself appears clear.

hands on: Actions actually performed by a caregiver.

health care proxy: Type of advanced directive in which the patient designates a person or persons to make their health care decisions for them if they are unable.

Heimlich maneuver: A procedure that is used to clear the windpipe of a person who is choking. It can be taught by local health promotion agencies.

hematological: Related to blood and its components.

high tech: Services or interventions requiring more extensive education of the caregiver and often special equipment. The delivery of home IV therapy is considered high tech.

home care agency: Agency that provides any or all services for the patient at home. Agencies that are not certified home health care agencies (CHHA) may have limited or restricted abilities and insurance coverage for them may vary.

home health aid (HHA): A person who provides hands on care to assist with or perform personal hygiene for the patient.

hospice: An agency designed to meet the specific needs of patients with terminal illness.

Hoyer lift: A mechanical, hydraulic device that is used to transfer the patient in and out of bed.

hydrotherapy: The use of water-based treatments, often whirlpool baths, to an affected body part or parts.

incontinence: Lack or reduction in the ability to control muscles related to urination and defecation.

incision: A cut made with a sharp tool, most often by a surgeon.

independence: The ability to perform activities unassisted.

infection: An invasion of the body by microorganisms that requires intervention.

inflammation: Localized redness, pain, heat and swelling.

instill: To apply drops, such as eye medication.

intervention: Action performed with a purpose to alter a situation.

intravenous: Delivery of medication directly into the blood stream through the use of a needle or catheter inserted into the vein.

lacerate: To tear or rip, usually unintentionally.

layperson: A person who has not received formal training.

lethargy: Drowsiness or slow response.

level of care: An assessment term whose definition and applications vary widely. Generally it's an indication of how extreme, intense or complicated the care for a patient is, or is anticipated to be.

limb: Refers to an arm or leg. This term is interchangeable with extremity.

living will: A form of advanced directive in which the patient states exactly which measures he or she would like to have implemented or omitted from care. Specific terms such as "no ventilator" or "no feeding tubes" are better interpreted than "no artificial means."

managed care: The practice of assigning a case manager or member of the health care team as a coordinator and primary resource for the patient. This is used in insurance and home care agencies.

manual dexterity: The ability to use the hands to perform a task efficiently and safely.

mechanical ventilation: Use of a ventilator to deliver oxygen into a patient's lung when the patient is unable to provide any or enough respiratory effort.

medical records: Records kept by each agency, hospital, facility or doctor regarding a patient's medical status, treatments, interventions and response.

medical status: The patient's current condition, diagnosis and level of functioning.

mobility: The action of moving about by ambulation or transfer.

mucous membranes: The surfaces of body channels that are exposed to air and contain mucous-secreting glands, such as the nose and mouth.

musculoskeletal (MS): Related to muscular and skeletal systems.

nailbeds: Area of the finger and toe under the nail surface. May be checked for cyanosis.

neurological: Related to the neurological system.

occupational therapy (OT): Professionally trained individuals who focus on rehabilitating the patient's self care abilities.

Office of the Aging: State-wide agencies that provide resources and interventions for the adult population. See appendix for list of offices of the aging in each state.

organ donor: A person who donates his or her organs for transplant, usually after death although some organs can be donated when the person is alive. The potential organ donor must make this wish known to his/her next-of-kin, however. Many hospitals will approach family members on the death of a patient who may be considered a likely organ donor.

orthopedic: Related to the joints, bones and associated muscles.

outpatient (OP): Services or treatments provided away from the patient's home, in a setting where the patient does not have to spend the night but can return home the same day.

over the counter (OTC): Medications that are available without a doctor's prescription.

palpitations: Heart beats that are felt by the patient, often described as flutters. May be a result of fatigue, caffeine use or related to medication or disease process.

pastoral counseling: A service provided by a specially-trained religious person to help explore and resolve some of the conflict and anxiety related to patient care, disease and illness.

per diem: Literally, "per day" in Latin. In home care, it refers to a health care worker who is employed by the day. A form of supplemental staffing.

perineal: Related to the skin, tissue and organs near the anus and vagina or penis.

physical therapy (PT): Professionally trained individuals who focus on rehabilitating the patient's muscle groups involved in ambulation and transfers.

PIC catheter: A peripherally inserted catheter, similar to a central venous catheter for the delivery of fluids or medication. It is inserted into one of the larger veins in the arm using sterile technique. It may be done at home by a specially trained nurse.

plateau: A level of functioning or rehabilitation where no more progress is anticipated. A plateau may be temporary until a change occurs in treatment (such as a cast removal) or until the patient recovers from an illness and his energy levels increase.

plunger: The end of a syringe where pressure is applied to inject a medication.

port a cath: A reservoir inserted under the skin with a catheter that is threaded into a large blood vessel near the heart. This procedure is done by a surgeon under sterile conditions. The port a cath is often placed on the chest wall. It is especially useful for patients who receive frequent medications such as chemotherapy, who receive medications that can irritate smaller veins, or who have blood drawn at regular intervals. The site is accessed by a needle through the skin that covers it, reducing the need for accessing veins in the arm.

prefill: Placing medications in a commercial or self-designed container for administration at prescribed intervals.

prescribed: Ordered by the doctor.

primary doctor: The doctor responsible for direction of the patients care.

purulent: A term used to describe drainage that is green, yellow or foul smelling, usually signaling an infection requiring intervention.

referral: Request for services of a particular agency or practitioner.

registered nurse (RN): Professionally trained individual who focuses on the treatment of disease and the restoration of health and well-being and the prevention of complications under the direction of a doctor.

rehabilitation: The act of restoring to previous or functional level.

secretions: Fluids and that are a natural and expected product of cell and body system function.

short of breath (SOB): Difficulty inhaling and/or exhaling as a symptom or result of a disease or illness.

social worker (SW or MSW): Professionally trained individual who acts to initiate or restore emotional, environmental and social well-being.

soft supplies: Disposable items used for patient care and treatment such as gloves, bandages, diapers.

speech therapy (ST): Professionally trained individuals who act to restore deficits in speech, and treat problems that pertain to the mouth and throat such as swallowing.

sphincter: A ring-like muscle that acts to close a body opening or passage.

stool: Feces.

suction: A mechanical device to remove excess secretions from a body cavity. may also be used when the patient is unable to naturally expel secretions.

supervision: To oversee and/or assist with an activity or action.

supply company: An agency that provides medical equipment and/or supplies; it may be contracted with a home care agency.

support group: Organized formal or informal gathering of individual with like concerns.

suppository: Medication in a solid tube-shaped base that is inserted either into the vagina or rectum delivery. May be used for anti nausea medications when a patient is vomiting.

syringe: A plastic tube to hold liquid medication for delivery which has a needle on one end for injection and a plunger on the other to perform the injection.

terminal: The stage of disease or illness when recovery is not expected or likely.

thickeners: Products available commercially that increase the thickness of liquids when swallowing is difficult.

tinnitus: Ringing in the ears. May be a result of medications or disease or a symptom.

total parenteral nutrition (TPN): Delivery of liquid nutrition intravenously that is individually formulated based on a patient's needs. It is used instead of, or in addition to, oral feedings. May be used as a life sustaining intervention or for a short period of time during recovery from surgery or illness.

tracheostomy: Incision into the trachea to allow insertion of a tube to facilitate breathing.

treatment: Intervention performed to improve recovery or treat an illness or symptom.

tub rail: Metal or heavy plastic tubing that is either installed directly onto the tub/shower walls or clamped onto the edge of the tub. Provides a sturdy grasping site to assist a patient who is using the tub or shower.

tubseat: A plastic bench or chair that is used inside the bathtub as a place for the patient to sit when bathing or showering.

underpad: Plastic-backed or heavy cloth pad that is placed under the patient to absorb body secretions and excess urine. Should not be the only method for urine collection for the incontinent patient unless directed by the nurse.

urethra: The canal through which urine is passed and exits the body.

urinary tract: Relates to the system for production and excretion of urine.

walker: A sturdy metal device with four legs and often wheels that provides support for a patient who is ambulating.

wheelchair: A device consisting of a seat, back and wheels which will move a patient for whom walking is not possible or is excessively tiring. May also be used to move a patient around in a home when otherwise unable.

wound care: The practice of cleaning a wound, applying a dressing or covering, and assessing the site. Initially this is done by a nurse and may be taught to the patient and/or family if appropriate. The doctor will provide orders for type and frequency of care to be provided.

18

ABBREVIATIONS

$\overline{a}$	before (*ante*)
ac	before meals (*ante cibum*)
AD	right ear (*auris dextra*)
ADL	activities of daily living
ad lib	as desired (*ad libitum*)
A.Fib	atrial fibrillation
AK	above knee
a.m.	before noon (*ante meridiem*)
AMA	against medical advice
amb	ambulate, ambulation
amt	amount
ant	anterior
ASCVD	arteriosclerotic cardiovascular disease
AS	left ear (*auris sinistra*)
ASHD	arteriosclerotic heart disease
AU	both ears (*auris unitas*)
AV	arteriovenous
bid	twice a day (*bis in die*)
bil	bilateral
biw	bi-weekly

BK	below knee
BM	bowel movement
BP	blood pressure
BPH	benign prostatic hypertrophy
BRP	bathroom privileges
BUN	blood urea nitrogen
$\bar{c}$	with (*cum*)
CA	cancer
Ca$^+$	calcium
CAD	coronary artery disease
CAT	computerized axial tomography
cath	catheter
CBC	complete blood count
CC	chief complaint
cc	cubic centimeter
CHHA	certified home health agency
CHF	congestive heart failure
Cl	chloride
CNS	central nervous system
C/O	complains of
CO$_2$	carbon dioxide
COPD	chronic obstructive pulmonary disease
CPR	cardiopulmonary resuscitation
C/S	culture and sensitivity
CVA	cerebrovascular accident
CXR	chest x-ray

D/C	discontinue
disch	discharge
DJD	degenerative joint disease
DM	diabetes mellitus
DNR	do not resuscitate
DOA	dead on arrival
DOB	date of birth
DSD	dry sterile dressing
DSS	Department of Social Service
Dx	diagnosis
ECG	electrocardiogram
EEG	electroencephalogram
EKG	electrocardiogram
ENT	ear, nose, throat
eval	evaluation
ext	extremity
FBS	fasting blood sugar
Fe	iron (*ferrum*)
Fe SO$_4$	iron sulfate
F/U	follow up
FUO	fever of unknown origin
FWB	full weight bearing
Fx	fracture
GB	gallbladder
GI	gastrointestinal
Gm	gram
gtt	drops (*guttae*)
GU	genitourinary

Gyn	gynecology
hct	hematocrit
HCVD	hypertensive cardiovascular disease
Hgb	hemoglobin
HHA	home health aid
HR	heart rate
HRF	health related facility
hs	at bedtime (*hora somni*)
HTN	hypertension
Hx	history
H$_2$O	water
IDDM	insulin dependent diabetes mellitus
IM	intramuscular
indep	independent
I&O	intake and output
K	thousand (*kilo*)
K+	potassium ion
L	left
LE	lower extremity
LQ	lower quadrant
LTC	long term care
MCR	Medicare
mg	milligram
Mg	magnesium
MI	myocardial infarction
min	minimal
MKD	medicaid
ml, mL	milliliter

mm	millimeter
mod	moderate
MS	multiple sclerosis
Na+	sodium
NG	nasogastric
NH	nursing home
NIDDM	non-insulin dependent diabetes mellitus
NKA	no known allergies
npo	nothing by mouth (*nil per os*)
NWB	non-weight bearing
O$_2$	oxygen
OA	osteoarthritis
OBS	organic brain syndrome
OD	right eye (*oculus dexter*)
od	every day (*omni die*)
OD	once a day
OOB	out of bed
OS	left eye (*oculus sinister*)
OT	occupational therapy
OU	both eyes (*oculi unitas*)
pc	after meals (*post cibum*)
PCG	personal caregiver
per	by
PERLA	pupils equal and reactive to light and accommodation
PHN	public health nurse
pm	afternoon (*post meridiem*)
PMH	past medical history
po	by mouth (*per os*)

pr	per rectum
prn	as needed (*pro re nata*)
PT	physical therapy
PTA	prior to admission
PWB	partial weight bearing
q	every (*quaque*)
qam	every morning
qh	every hour (*quaque hora*)
q2h	every 2 hours
q3h	every 3 hours
qid	four times a day (*quater in die*) 10am, 2pm, 6pm, 10pm
R	right
RA	rheumatoid arthritis
reg	regular
RBC	red blood (cell) count
re	regarding
R/O	rule out
ROM	range of motion
RR	respiratory rate
RN	registered nurse
Rx	prescription
s.e.	side effects
SL	sublingual, under the tongue (*sub lingua*)
SN	skilled nursing
SNF	skilled nursing facility
SOB	shortness of breath
s/p	status post
S&S, S/S	signs and symptoms

ST	speech therapy
stat	immediately (*statim*)
Sx	signs, symptoms
tabs	tablets
temp	temperature
tbsp	tablespoon
T/C	telephone call
TIA	transient ischemic attack
tid	three times a day (*ter in die*)
TPR	temperature, pulse and respiration
TURP	transurethral resection of prostate
tsp	teaspoon
U/A	urinalysis
UE	upper extremity
URI	upper respiratory infection
UTI	urinary tract infection
VNS	visiting nurse service
vol	volume
VS	vital signs
WBC	white blood (cell) count
w/c	wheelchair
WNL	within normal limits
X	times

MEASUREMENTS

1 cup = 8 fl oz = 16 Tbsp = 48 tsp = 237 ml

3/4 cup = 6 fl oz = 12 Tbsp = 36 tsp = 177 ml

2/3 cup = 5 1/3 fl oz = 10 2/3 Tbsp = 32 tsp = 158 ml

1/2 cup = 4 fl oz = 8 Tbsp = 24 tsp = 118 ml

1/3 cup = 2 2/3 fl oz = 5 1/3 Tbsp = 16 tsp = 79 ml

1/4 cup = 2 fl oz = 4 Tbsp = 12 tsp = 59 ml

1/8 cup = 1 fl oz = 2 Tbsp = 6 tsp = 30 ml

1 Tbsp = 3 tsp = 15 ml

1 tsp = 5 ml

MEDICATION TIMES

The following list for nonprofessional caregivers is an interpretation of certain abbreviations related to medication administration. These are only a guideline. Actual orders should be verified with the doctor, and times should be adapted to the patient's routine with regard to the time that he wakes, has his meals or goes to bed.

OD   once a day (10 a.m.)

bid   twice a day (10 a.m. and 6 p.m.)

tid   three times a day (10 a.m., 2 p.m., 6 p.m.)

hs   at bedtime (10 p.m.)

qid   four times a day (10 a.m., 2 p.m., 6 p.m., 10 p.m.)

19

RESOURCES

Resources are available for almost every medical condition, disease process, and social need. The first step in obtaining the best information is to have the doctor write down the patient's diagnosis. A verbal diagnosis is often misinterpreted and may lead to the accumulation of incorrect information.

Keep a folder in an accessible location. This provides a place in which to accumulate all the information that is gathered. When an article, phone number or any other pertinent information is found, place it in the folder. Being aware of current studies, usual interventions or alternative treatments can make patient care easier, or at least make more sense. The information can be copied and forwarded to all family/advocates involved in care. This will help keep them abreast of what treatment or intervention is needed or suggested.

NATIONAL DISEASE ORGANIZATIONS

Once a diagnosis is made, or a medical condition is documented, you may start by contacting its local or national foundation. The phone book may have listings for such organizations as the American Cancer Society or the American Heart Association. If the phone book does not have listings, the "800" number directory (1-800-555-1212) may be able to provide a phone number. In the event that there is not a toll-free number, you may call the local hospital discharge planning department or social service department, which should have the numbers.

When calling such organizations, they may ask about the patient's diagnosis, when it was made, as well as the patient's name and address. The diagnosis information is not necessarily attached to the patient's record, but may be used for statistical information by the organization. It may send disease-specific information to the patient, such as pamphlets explaining how the disease occurs and current trends in care. It may also be able to provide a list of doctors and treatment centers in the patient's geographical area.

SUPPORT GROUPS

Support groups pertaining to the disease are another way to obtain information, as well as a way to network with patients and caregivers. Support groups may be found through the doctor's office, religious groups, posted message centers in the community or hospital, or on the internet.

Support groups or local chapters of disease-related groups may provide information regarding local doctors who specialize in the treatment of the disease, hospitals providing the most aggressive or current treatments, and any experimental treatments or studies that are being conducted.

Please note that internet sites may change frequently. Those provided were updated in June, 1998.

LISTINGS

Alzheimers Association
1-800-272-3900
Web site: http://www.alz.org

American Association of Geriatric Psychiatry
1-301-654-7850
Web site: http://www.aagpgpa.org

American Association of Retired Persons
1-800-424-3410
Web site: http://www.aarp.org

American Cancer Society
1-800-227-2345
Web site: http://www.cancer.org

American Diabetes Association
1-800-342-2383
Web site: http://www.diabetes.org

American Heart Association
1-800-242-8721
Web site: http://www.amhrt.org

American Lung Association
1-800-586-4872
Web site: http://www.lungusa.org/index.html

Arthritis Foundation
1-800-283-7800
Web site: http://www.arthritis.org

Cancer information Service, National Cancer Institute
1-800-422-6237
Web site: http://www.nci.nih.gov

CDC National AIDS Clearinghouse
1-800-458-5231
Web site: http://www.cdcnac.org

Children of Aging Parents
1-800-227-7294
Web site: access at http://www.careguide.com

Elderweb
Web site: http://www.elderweb.com

Family Caregivers Alliance
1-800-445-8106
Web site: http://www.caregiver.org

Grief Recovery Helpline,
The Grief Recovery Institute Educational Foundation Inc.
1-800-445-4808
Web site: http://www.grief-recovery.com

Health Insurance Association of America
1-202-824-1600
Web site: http://www.hiaa.org

Homecare America
1-877-SHOP-HCA (call for store location)
Web site: http://www.homecareamerica.com

Homecare on the Internet
Web site: http://www.homecare.org

Hospice Education Institute
1-800-331-1620
E-Mail: HospiceAll@aol.com

Medic Alert
1-800-825-3785
Web site: http://www.medicalert.org

National Association for Continence
1-800-252-3337
Web site: http://www.nafc.org

National Association of Area Agencies for the Aging/Eldercare Locator
1-800-677-1116
Web site: http://www.n4A.org

National Family Caregivers Association
1-800-896-3650
Web site: http://www.nfcacares.org

National Institute of Aging Information Center, National Institute on Aging
1-800-222-2225
Web site: http://www.nih.gov/nia/

National Stroke Association
1-800-787-6537
Web site: http://www.stroke.org

Office of Minority Health Resource Center, Office of Minority Health
1-800-444-6472
Web site: http://www.omhrc.gov

Social Security Administration
1-800-772-1213
Web site: http://www.ssa.gov

Spinal Cord Injury Network
1-800-548-2673
Web site: http://www.sonic.net/spinal/

U.S. Administration on Aging, Department of Health and Human Services
1-202-619-0724
Web site: http://www.aoa.dhhs.gov

Visiting Nurse Association of America
1-800-426-2547
Web site: http://www.Vnaa.org

20

JUST FOR SENIORS

SENIOR CITIZEN GROUPS

Local senior citizen groups may provide "friendly caller" services that assign a patient to a caller who checks in with the patient via telephone on a regular basis. There is usually a backup plan in place in case a patient does not answer as planned. For example, a neighbor, family member or friend might then be called. The caller may just "check in" with the patient, or may remind the patient to take medications or keep appointments. The patient must have a phone and be able to answer it in order for this service to be productive.

Local high schools sometimes organize the students to provide community services such as raking leaves, grocery shopping, or taking the patient for a walk. A call to the school's guidance counselor can determine what services may be available. High school students are sometimes available as volunteers or for-hire at set rates to perform such tasks as taking out a patient's garbage, tending the garden, raking leaves, mowing the lawn or shoveling snow. Students may also be able to do light housekeeping, deliver groceries or keep the patient company, read to them or assist with letter writing.

There are many sources of information and assistance available. Patients should be encouraged to use all available services.

OFFICES OF THE AGING

Most cities and/or counties have organized offices of the aging that offer programs and services for the elderly. These offices are also able to make referrals for needs that they cannot meet. The following is a short list of some of the services that they can provide.

Health Screenings

Offices of the aging often sponsor blood pressure and other screenings that are open to the public. A nurse is usually stationed at an accessible location in the community, such as a library or senior citizen meeting place. The nurse can also discuss basic health care, nutrition and medication administration. Patients who need more specific information may decide that they need to see a doctor or be referred for visiting nurse services. Such screenings are important because they can help identify potential medical problems. Similar services are also provided by health care and government agencies.

Meal Delivery

Offices of the aging can direct senior citizens to programs that deliver balanced meals, hot or cold, to the home for a reasonable fee. Some groups provide Kosher meals, but most cannot accommodate rigid diet restrictions such as low fat or no salt; check with the organization beforehand. In addition to bringing the meals, the volunteer for the organization also provides some limited socialization for the patient.

Social Events

Scheduled social events, such as museum and shopping trips, get senior citizens out of the house and allow them to interact with their peers. Check for hidden costs such as lodging or meals. Special interest groups that provide trips not only allow for interaction, but put seniors in touch with others who have similar interests. If medications need to be taken while out on a trip, be sure to bring them in a medication box that is securely sealed and marked with the person's name. Bottled water can be carried along for use with medication.

Classes and Workshops

Workshops can help senior citizens familiarize themselves with their legal rights to elder services, insurance benefits, etc. These workshops can also assist the person in obtaining other entitlements such as property tax breaks for senior citizens. Additional classes focus on enhancing physical strength or emotional well-being.

Social Workers

A social worker may be available through the office of the aging to help a patient obtain needed services, such as senior housing, subsidized food purchase, or the services of an attorney who specializes in elder law. Social workers can also provide information regarding how to deal with insurance companies, including how to dispute an insurance claim, how to investigate non-payment on a claim or how to contact an insurance company to arrange for monthly payments of an insurance bill.

Home Repair

Offices of the aging can provide referrals for home repair and maintenance service, from changing a light bulb to cleaning gutters. Some services are provided by other senior citizens for a small fees or on a volunteer basis; others may be provided by local high school students or religious groups.

Volunteer Activities

Offices of the aging may be able to arrange for the patient to participate in volunteer activities, such as knitting hats for a local hospital nursery. Patients who participate in volunteer activities and give something of themselves back to others will find their feelings of self esteem and independence enhanced. This contributes to better mental and physical well being, as well as healing.

STATE LISTINGS

Alabama
Martha Murph Beck, Executive Director
Alabama Commission on Aging
RSA Plaza, Suite 470
770 Washington Avenue
Montgomery, AL 36130-0001
(334) 242-5743
FAX: (334)242-5594
Web site: http://webserver.dsmd.state.al.us/COA/

Alaska
Kay Burrows, Acting Director
Alaska Commission on Aging, Division of Senior Services
Department of Administration
3601 C Street, #310
Anchorage, AK 99503-5209
(907) 269-3666
FAX: (907) 269-3690
Web site: http://www.state.ak.us/local/akpages/ADMIN/dss/homess.htm

Arizona
Henry Blanco, Acting Administrator
Aging and Adult Administration
Department of Economic Security
1789 West Jefferson-#950A
Phoenix, AZ 85007-3202
(602) 542-4446
FAX: (602) 542-6575
Web site: www.DESAA.primenet.com

Arkansas
Herb Sanderson, Director
Division of Aging and Adult Services
Arkansas Dept. of Human Services
P.O. Box 1437, Slot 1412

Little Rock, AR 72203-1437
(501) 682-2441
FAX: (501) 682-8155
Web site: http://www.state.ar.us/dhs/index2.html

California
Dixon Arnette, Director
California Department of Aging
1600 K Street
Sacramento, CA 95814-4020
(916) 322-4383
FAX: (916) 322-1903
Web site: http://www.aging.state.ca.us/

Colorado
Rita Barreras, Director
Aging and Adult Services
Department of Human Services
110-16th Street, Suite 200
Denver, CO 80202-5202
(303) 620-4147
FAX: (303) 620-4189
Web site: http://www.state.co.us/gov_dir/human_services_dir/
AAS/index.htm

Connecticut
Christine M. Lewis, Director of Community Services
Division of Elderly Services
25 Sigourney Street
Hartford, CT 06106-5033
1-800-443-9946 within CT
(860) 424-4925 Out of state
FAX: (860) 424-4966
Web site: http://www.dss.state.ct.us/svcs/elderly.htm

Delaware
Eleanor Cain, Director
Delaware Department of Health and Social Services
Division of Services for Aging and Adults with Physical Disabilities
1901 North DuPont Highway
New Castle, DE 19720-1100
(302) 577-4791
FAX: (302) 577-4793
Web site: http://kidshealth.org/nhc/divage/index.html

District of Columbia
E. Veronica Pace, Executive Director
District of Columbia Office on Aging
441 Fourth Street, N.W., Suite 900 South
Washington, DC 20001-2714
(202) 724-5622
FAX: (202) 724-4979
Web site: http://www.ci.washington.dc.us/AGING/aghome.htm

Florida
Bentley Lipscomb, Secretary
Department of Elder Affairs
4040 Esplanade Way
Tallahassee, FL 32399-7000
(850) 414-2000
FAX: (850) 414-2002
Web site: http://fcn.state.fl.us/doea/doea.html

Georgia
Judy Hagebak, Director
Division of Aging Services
Department of Human Resources
2 Peachtree Street NW, Suite 36-385
Atlanta, GA 30303-3104
(404) 657-5258
FAX: (404) 657-5285
Web site: http://www.state.ga.us/Departments/DHR/aging.html

Hawaii
Marilyn Seely, Director
Hawaii Executive Office on Aging
No. 1 Capitol District
250 South Hotel Street, Room 109
Honolulu, HI 96813-2831
(808) 586-0100
FAX: (808) 586-0815
Web site: http://www.maui.net/~cristan/

Idaho
Arlene Davidson, Director
Idaho Commission on Aging
700 W. Jefferson-P.O. Box 83720-0007, Room 108
Boise, ID 83720-0007
(208) 334-3833
FAX: (208) 334-3033
Web site: http://www2.state.id.us/icoa/

Illinois
Maralee Lindley, Director
Illinois Department on Aging
421 East Capitol Avenue, Suite 100
Springfield, IL 62701-1789
(217) 785-3356
FAX: (217) 785-4477
Chicago Office: (312) 814-2630
Web site: http://www.state.il.us/aging/

Indiana
Geneva Shedd, Director
Family and Social Services Administration
Division of Disability, Aging and Rehabilitative Services
Bureau of Aging and In-Home Services
402 W. Washington Street, #W454
Indianapolis, IN 46207-7083

(317) 232-7020
FAX: (317) 232-7867
Web site: http://www.drugs.indiana.edu/indiana/fssa.html#DDARS

Iowa
Betty Grandquist, Executive Director
Department of Elder Affairs
Celemens Building, 3rd Floor
200 Tenth Street
Des Moines, IA 50309-3609
(515) 281-5188
FAX: (515) 281-4036
Web site: http://www.sos.state.ia.us/register/r4/r4eldaf.htm

Kansas
Thelma Hunter Gordon, Secretary
Kansas Department on Aging
New England Building
503 South Kansas
Topeka, KS 66603-3404
(913) 296-4986
FAX: (913) 296-0256
Web site: http://www.K4s.org/kdoa/default.htm

Kentucky
Jerry Whitley, Director
Kentucky Division of Aging Services
Cabinet for Human Resources
275 East Main Street, 5 West
Frankfort, KY 40621-0001
(502) 564-6930
FAX: (502) 564-4595
Web site: No site available

Louisiana
P.F. "Pete" Arceneaux, Director
Governor's Office of Elderly Affairs
P.O. Box 80374
412 N 4th Street
Baton Rouge, LA 70802-5523
(504) 342-7100
FAX: (504) 342-7133
Web site: no site available

Maine
Christine Gianopoulos, Director
Bureau of Elder and Adult Services
Department of Human Services
35 Anthony Avenue
11 State House Station
Augusta, ME 04333-0001
(207) 624-5335
FAX: (207) 624-5361
Web site: http://www.state.me.us/beas/dhs_beas.htm

Maryland
Sue Ward, Director
Maryland Office on Aging
State Office Building, Room 1007
301 West Preston Street
Baltimore, MD 21201-2374
(410) 767-1100
FAX: (410) 333-7943
Web site: http://www.inform.umd.edu/UMS+State/MD_Resources/
OOA/index.html

Massachusetts
Lillian Glickman, Acting Secretary
Massachusetts Executive Office of Elder Affairs
One Ashburton Place, 5th Floor
Boston, MA 02108-1518
(617) 727-7750
FAX: (617) 727-9368
Web site: http://www.magnet.state.ma.us/bb/fy97h1/eoea.htm

Michigan
Lynn Alexander, Director
Office of Services to the Aging
P.O. Box 30676
Lansing, MI 48909-8176
(517) 373-8230
FAX: (517) 373-4092
Web site: http://www.mass.iog.wayne.edu/MASShome.html

Minnesota
James G. Varpness, Executive Secretary
Minnesota Board on Aging
444 Lafayette Road
St. Paul, MN 55155-3843
(612) 296-2770
FAX: (612) 297-7855
Web site: http://www.dhs.state.mn.us

Mississippi
Eddie Anderson, Director
Division of Aging and Adult Services
750 N. State Street
Jackson, MS 39202-3033
(601) 359-4929
FAX: (601) 359-4370
Web site: http://www.mdhs.state.ms.us/aas.html

Missouri

Andrea J. Routh, Director

Division on Aging

Department of Social Services

P.O. Box 1337

65109 Howerton Court

Jefferson City, MO 65102-1337

(573) 751-3082

FAX: (573) 751-8687

Web site: http://www.state.mo.us/dss/da/da.htm

Montana

Charles Rehbein, Bureau Chief

Senior and Long Term Care Division

Department of Public Health and Human Services

P.O. Box 4210

Helena, MT 59604-4210

(406) 444-4077

FAX: (406) 444-7743

Web site: http://www.dphhs.mt.gov

Nebraska

Mark Intermill, Administrator

Department of Health and Human Services

Division on Aging

P.O. Box 95044

301 Centennial Mall South

Lincoln, NE 68509-5044

(402) 471-2307

FAX: (402) 471-4619

Web site: http://www.hhs.state.ne.us/

Nevada

Carla Sloane, Administrator

Nevada Division for Aging Services

Department of Human Resources

340 North 11th Street, Suite 203

Las Vegas, NV 89101-3125
(702) 486-3545
FAX: (702) 486-3572
Web site: http://www.state.nv.us/hr/aging/

New Hampshire
Catherine A. Keane, Interim Director
Division of Elderly and Adult Services
State Office Park South
115 Pleasant Street, Annex Bldg. #1
Concord, NH 03301-3843
(603) 271-4680
FAX: (603) 271-4643
Web site: http://www.state.nh.us/dhhs/ofs/ofscstlc.htm

New Jersey
Ruth Reader, Assistant Commissioner
Department of Health and Senior Services
Division of Senior Affairs
Quaker Bridge Road
Quaker Bridge Plaza #12B
Hamilton Township, NJ 08619
1-800 792-8820 within NJ
(609) 588-3392 Out of state
FAX: (609) 633-6609
Web site: http://www.state.nj.us/health

New Mexico
Michelle Lujan Grisham, Director
State Agency on Aging
La Villa Rivera Building
228 East Palace Avenue
Santa Fe, NM 87501-2013
(505) 827-7640
FAX: (505) 827-7649
Web site: No site available

New York
Walter G. Hoefer, Executive Director
New York State Office for The Aging
2 Empire State Plaza
Albany, NY 12223-1251
1-800-342-9871 Within NY
(518) 474-5731 Outside NY
FAX: (518) 474-0608
Web site: http://www. aging.state.ny.us/nysofa

North Carolina
Karen E. Gottovi, Director
Division of Aging
CB 29531
693 Palmer Drive
Raleigh, NC 27626-0531
(919) 733-3983
FAX: (919) 733-0443
Web site: http://www.state.nc.us/DHR/DOA/home.htm

North Dakota
Linda Wright, Director
Department of Human Services
Aging Services Division
600 South 2nd Street, Suite 1C
Bismarck, ND 58504-5729
(701) 328-8910
FAX: (701) 328-8989
Web site: No site available

Ohio
Judith Y. Brachman, Director
Ohio Department of Aging
50 West Broad Street-9th Floor
Columbus, OH 43215-5928

(614) 466-5500
FAX: (614) 466-5741
Web site: http://www.state.oh.us/Y2K10Y2Kage.html

Oklahoma
Roy R. Keen, Division Administrator
Services for the Aging
Department of Human Services
P.O. Box 25352
312 N.E. 28th Street
Oklahoma City, OK 73105-2804
(405) 521-2281 or 521-2327
FAX: (405) 521-2086
Web site: http://www.onenet.net/okdhs/division/aging/sooa.htm

Oregon
Roger Auerbach, Administrator
Senior and Disabled Services Division
500 Summer Street, N.E., 2nd Floor
Salem, OR 97310-1015
(503) 945-5811
FAX: (503) 373-7823
Web site: http://www.sdsd.hr.state.or.us/

Pennsylvania
Richard Browdie, Secretary
Pennsylvania Department of Aging
Commonwealth of Pennsylvania
555 Walnut Street, 5th Floor
Harrisburg, PA 17101-1919
(717) 783-1550
FAX: (717) 783-6842
Web site: http://164.156.7.66/PA_Exec/Aging/overview.html

Rhode Island
Barbara Rayner, Director
Department of Elderly Affairs
160 Pine Street
Providence, RI 02903-3708
(401) 222-2858
FAX: (401) 222-1490
Web site: http://www.sec.state.ri.us:80/STDEPT/sd23.htm

South Carolina
Constance C. Rinehart, Deputy Director
Office on Aging
South Carolina Department of Health and Human services
P.O. Box 8206
Columbia, SC 29202-8206
(803) 253-6177
FAX: (803) 253-4173
Web site: http://agweb.clemson.edu/Fin/comage.htm

South Dakota
Gail Ferris, Administrator
Office of Adult Services and Aging
Richard F. Kneip Building
700 Governors Drive
Pierre, SD 57501-2291
(605) 773-3656
FAX: (605) 773-6834
Web site: http://www.state.sd.us/state/executive/social/ASA.htm

Tennessee
James S. Whaley, Executive Director
Commission on Aging
Andrew Jackson Building, 9th Floor
500 Deaderick Street
Nashville, TN 37243-0860
(615) 741-2056
FAX: (615) 741-3309

Web site: http://www.state.tn.us/health/nhrgap
(site relates to state "health gap" program)

Texas
Mary Sapp, Executive Director
Texas Department on Aging
4900 North Lamar, 4th Floor
P.O.Box 12786
Austin, TX 78751-2316
(512) 424-6840
FAX: (512) 424-6890
Web site: http://www.tdoa.state.tx.us/index.htm

Utah
Helen Goddard, Division Director
Division of Aging & Adult Services
Box 45500
Salt Lake City, UT 84145-0500
(801) 538-3910
FAX: (801) 538-4395
Web site: http://www.dhs.state.ut.us/

Vermont
David Yavocone, Commissioner
Vermont Department of Aging and Disabilities
Waterbury Complex
103 South Main Street
Waterbury VT 05671-2301
(802) 241-2400
FAX: (802) 241-2325
Web site: http://www.state.vt.us/dad/index.html

Virginia
Dr. Ann McGee, Director
Virginia Department for the Aging
1600 Forest Avenue, Suite 102
Richmond, VA 23229-5007

1-800-552-3402 within VA
(804) 662-9333 out of state
FAX: (804) 662-9354
Web site: http://www.Aging.state.va.us

Washington

Ralph Smith, Assistant Secretary
Aging and Adult Services Administration
Department of Social and Health Services
P.O. Box 45050
Olympia, WA 98504-5050
(360) 586-8753
FAX: (360) 902-7848
Web site: http://www.wa.gov/dshs/administrations.html#aasa

West Virginia

Patricia F. Bradford, Commissioner
West Virginia Bureau of Senior Services
Holly Grove-State Capitol
1900 Kanawha Boulevard East
Charleston, WV 25305-0160
(304) 558-3317
FAX: (304) 558-0004
Web site: http://www.wvdhhr.org/pages/bcs/aging.htm

Wisconsin

Donna McDowell, Director
Bureau of Aging and Long Term Care Resources
Department of Health and Family Services
P.O. Box 7851
Madison, WI 53707-7851
(608) 266-2536
FAX: (608) 267-3203
Web site: http://www.dhfs.state.wi.us/

Wyoming
Edna Vajda, Program Manager
Office on Aging
Department of Health
117 Hathaway Building, Room 139
Cheyenne, WY 82002-0480
(307) 777-7986
FAX: (307) 777-5340
Web site: no site available

INDEX

ABOUT THE AUTHOR

For the past 10 years, Ellen M. Caruso, R.N., has been helping patients make the transition from hospital to home care. As a visiting nurse, she has provided countless concerned family members and caregivers with the information they need to create a safe and healthy environment for the patient in the home.

Caruso's nursing career includes experience in intensive care, experimental HIV drug therapy, hi-tech infusion, and case management. She has also supervised home health workers and nursing staff.

She is a graduate of the Cochran School of Nursing, in Yonkers, New York and is a member of National Family Caregivers Association. Caruso lives with her husband and two sons in Poughkeepsie, New York.